T0054472

GROW A NEW BODY

Also by Alberto Villoldo

THE HEART OF THE SHAMAN:
Stories and Practices of the Luminous Warrior*

MYSTICAL SHAMAN ORACLE
(with Marcela Lobos and Colette Baron-Reid)*

POWER UP YOUR BRAIN: The Neuroscience of Enlightenment
(with David Perlmutter, M.D., F.A.C.N.)*

THE ILLUMINATION PROCESS: A Shamanic Guide to
Transforming Toxic Emotions into Wisdom, Power, and Grace*

COURAGEOUS DREAMING:
How Shamans Dream the World into Being*

YOGA, POWER, AND SPIRIT: Pantanjali the Shaman*

THE FOUR INSIGHTS:
Wisdom, Power, and Grace of the Earthkeepers*

SOUL JOURNEYING: Shamanic Tools for
Finding Your Destiny and Recovering Your Spirit *

SHAMAN, HEALER, SAGE: How to Heal Yourself and Others with
the Energy Medicine of the Americas

DANCE OF THE FOUR WINDS:
Secrets of the Inca Medicine Wheel (with Erik Jendresen)

ISLAND OF THE SUN:
Mastering the Inca Medicine Wheel (with Erik Jendresen)

*Available from Hay House

Please visit:

Hay House USA: www.hayhouse.com®
Hay House Australia: www.hayhouse.com.au
Hay House UK: www.hayhouse.co.uk
Hay House India: www.hayhouse.co.in

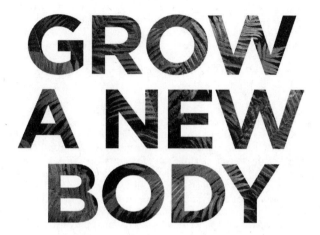

GROW A NEW BODY

How Spirit and Power Plant Nutrients Can Transform Your Health

Dr. Alberto Villoldo

HAY HOUSE, INC.
Carlsbad, California • New York City
London • Sydney • New Delhi

Copyright © 2019 by Alberto Villoldo

Published in the United States by: Hay House, Inc.: www.hayhouse.com® • *Published in Australia by:* Hay House Australia Pty. Ltd.: www.hayhouse.com.au
Published in the United Kingdom by: Hay House UK, Ltd.: www.hayhouse.co.uk
Published in India by: Hay House Publishers India: www.hayhouse.co.in

Cover design: Barbara LeVan Fisher • *Interior design:* Nick C. Welch

All rights reserved. No part of this book may be reproduced by any mechanical, photographic, or electronic process, or in the form of a phonographic recording; nor may it be stored in a retrieval system, transmitted, or otherwise be copied for public or private use—other than for "fair use" as brief quotations embodied in articles and reviews—without prior written permission of the publisher.

The author of this book does not dispense medical advice or prescribe the use of any technique as a form of treatment for physical, emotional, or medical problems without the advice of a physician, either directly or indirectly. The intent of the author is only to offer information of a general nature to help you in your quest for emotional, physical, and spiritual well-being. In the event you use any of the information in this book for yourself, the author and the publisher assume no responsibility for your actions.

To protect the privacy of others, certain names and details have been changed.

Portions of this book were previously published by Hay House as *One Spirit Medicine* © Alberto Villoldo (hardcover 978-1-4019-4730-9, tradepaper 978-1-4019-4731-6)

Library of Congress Cataloging-in-Publication Data

Names: Villoldo, Alberto, author.
Title: Grow a new body : how spirit and power plant nutrients can transform your health / Alberto Villoldo.
Other titles: One spirit medicine
Description: Carlsbad, California : Hay House Inc., [2019] | Revision of: One spirit medicine. 2014.
Identifiers: LCCN 2018049678| ISBN 9781401956561 (paperback) | ISBN 9781401956578 (ebook) | ISBN 9781401956738 (audiobook)
Subjects: LCSH: Spiritual healing--Shamanism. | Shamanism. | Medicine, Magic, mystic, and spagiric. | Health. | BISAC: BODY, MIND & SPIRIT / Healing / General. | HEALTH & FITNESS / Alternative Therapies. | BODY, MIND & SPIRIT / Spirituality / Shamanism.
Classification: LCC BF1623.S63 V55 2019 | DDC 131--dc23 LC record available at https://lccn.loc.gov/2018049678

Tradepaper ISBN: 978-1-4019-5656-1
e-book ISBN: 978-1-4019-5657-8
Audiobook ISBN: 978-1-4019-5673-8

16 15 14 13 12 11 10 9 8 7
1st edition, March 2019

Printed in the United States of America

To Patty Gift,
with love and eternal gratitude

CONTENTS

Part V: The Grow a New Body Program

INTRODUCTION

The Gifts of One Spirit Medicine

You can grow a new body. You know you can, because you have *already* grown a body once before. Ten fingers, ten toes, all of the exquisite beauty of your physique grew from an egg and a sperm following careful instructions. And to grow a *new* body, all you have to do is break in to the password-protected regions of your DNA to switch on these same codes.

I know this is possible because I did it.

You see, I had no choice.

At the time of this incident, everything was going well for me. Professionally I was at the top of my game, a best-selling author with 12 books to my credit, a medical anthropologist with a Ph.D. in psychology, a teacher and healer with a following worldwide. The Four Winds Society that I founded had grown exponentially: more than 5,000 students had gone through our training in energy medicine or had accompanied me on journeys to the Amazon and the Andes. And those were just the accomplishments the public could see. Close to my heart were the many inner gifts I had received on my journey, including the most precious gift of all, a beloved partner who walks a spirited path beside me.

Just when it looked as if life couldn't get any better, I was stopped in my tracks. Suddenly I was in a fight for survival that called on everything I'd learned in 30 years of studying with some of the world's most gifted healers. You see, I am trained in neuroscience but I am also a shaman, initiated in the healing ways of the indigenous peoples I studied in the jungles and mountains of South America.

Clearly the Amazon rain forest is not the Beverly Hilton, so when I tell people what I do, they often say, "Are you nuts?" I understand their concern. The way of the shaman is not for everyone. The training is rigorous and demanding, and my extended stays in the jungle exacted a heavy price.

While I was in Mexico as a keynote speaker at a conference on science and consciousness, without warning I found I couldn't walk 100 feet without collapsing in exhaustion. Friends chalked it up to my crazy travel schedule, but I knew something was terribly wrong.

A few days before the trip I had gone for a head-to-toe checkup, a complete battery of tests from medical specialists in Miami. I got my test results in Mexico; the news was not good. Apparently, during my years of research in Indonesia, Africa, and South America, I had picked up a long list of nasty microorganisms, including five different kinds of hepatitis virus, three or four varieties of deadly parasites, and a host of toxic bacteria. My heart and liver were close to collapse, the doctors said, and my brain was riddled with parasites.

When I heard the words, "It's your brain, Dr. Villoldo," I sank into despair. The irony was I had just published a book entitled *Power Up Your Brain: The Neuroscience of Enlightenment*. The doctors advised me to get my name on a liver transplant list. Maybe my heart would recover, but where was I going to find a healthy brain?

After the conference, my wife, Marcela, was going on to the Amazon to lead one of our expeditions through The Four Winds Society. I stood in the departure wing at the Cancún airport, staring at my options: Gate 15, the flight to Miami where I would be admitted to a top medical center, or Gate 14, the flight to Lima and the Amazon, where I would be with Marcela in the land of my spiritual roots. All my test results indicated I was dying. Miami was the logical choice. I boarded the plane and eased into my seat. Just as the flight attendant offered me a moist towel, a primal instinct made me sit bolt upright and summon up the courage to put my future where my mouth was—to live what I had taught to so many. My journal entry for that night reads:

> *I knew I had to go to the jungle. Otherwise I would be looking for my medicine in the wrong place. Now I am with the woman I love, returning to the garden where I first found my spiritual path.*

In the Amazon, the shamans welcomed me lovingly. These men and women were friends who had known me for decades. And who knew me better than Mother Earth? She received me as only a mother can. As I pressed my body to hers, I felt her speak to me: "Welcome home, my son."

That night there was a ceremony with a brew made from the *Banisteriopsis caapi* vine that shamans use for visioning and healing. I was too weak to participate, so I stayed in our cottage by the river. Marcela went to the ceremony for both of us. I could hear the shaman whistling, and his haunting songs wafted across the water to me as I went into a light meditation.

Hours later Marcela returned smiling. Mother Earth had spoken to her that night: "I make everything on the earth grow. I am giving Alberto a new liver. He knows how to heal everything else." The next day I wrote in my journal:

> *After morning yoga, a being appeared to me in broad daylight. She walked out of the river, and I saw her as if in a dream—a spirit who touched my chest and told me that I was a child of the Pachamama and that she would look after me, as my work on the earth is not yet done.*

My return to the Amazon was the beginning of my healing. But first there was an enormous amount of work to do. I was gravely ill. I had to hack my biology to switch on the genes that create health and that would help me to grow a new brain, a new heart, and a new liver. And I had to remind myself: *There are no guarantees, Alberto. There is a difference between curing and healing.*

You may not be cured; you may die. But regardless of what happens, your soul will be healed.

From the Amazon, Marcela and I flew to Chile and our Center for Energy Medicine near Mount Aconcagua, the highest peak in the Americas. In the Inka language, *aconcagua* means "where you come to meet God." This is exactly what I needed. It was time for the meeting I had been postponing for so long.

My body was a road map of the jungles and mountains where I had worked as an anthropologist, picking up the lethal critters that had taken up residence inside me. The jungle is a living biology laboratory, and if you spend enough time there, you become part of the experiment. I knew anthropologists who had died of the parasites I now harbored.

Actually, the virgin rain forest of the Amazon is free of most disease, but to get to it you have to go through filth-ridden outposts of Western civilization. The Indios knew better than to foul their nests and their drinking water. Meanwhile, the white man surrounded himself with a sea of garbage and sewage.

The spiritual medicine I received from the shamans when I was in the Amazon was powerful, but I had to complement it with Western science. The doctors put me on a worm medication—the same type I give my dogs—and on antibiotics to kill other parasites. My brain was on fire with inflammatory agents produced by the medications and the dead and dying parasites. I would have to detox my brain to avoid going completely mad.

My brain fog and confusion were glaringly evident when I tried to play *Scrabble* with Marcela. That game became the barometer of my mental health. I could not access words. And then I started losing my sense of self. I panicked: *What if I forget who I am? What if I lose my awareness of self?* Madness stared at me from the horizon—I saw it, felt it, breathed it. It sent naked fear into every part of my being.

Ironically, it was fear of losing myself that saved me: over the next three months, I simply observed the madness I was experiencing. The Buddhists have a powerful practice of self-inquiry that starts with asking, *Who am I?* Then, after a while, you begin to inquire, *Who is it who is asking the question?* So I began to ask, *Who is it who's going mad?*

There was no place to hide. I saw the madness; others saw it. But, as always, there was another side to the pain. The fathomless depths to which my spirit sank were matched by the flight of my soul. I began to understand who I had been since the beginning of time and who I would be after I died. The gnawing fear was matched by divine love and a dawning experience of Oneness I had never felt before.

I called my friend David Perlmutter, a neurologist who was the co-author of my book *Power Up Your Brain.* Together we crafted a strategy using potent antioxidants and extreme ketosis (where the body uses fats instead of sugars as fuel) to trigger the production of neural stem cells to repair my brain. Over the next three months, I began to understand how unhealed emotions create disease, and how I had to heal my anger and my fear in order to recover my health. Energy moved, flowed, met obstacles, and flowed again. Time drifted by like a sluggish river, and I stepped out of it, knowing I had to make friends with eternity.

That night, I had a dream:

I am with friends looking at a grave covered with flowers. I am buried there. My friends say I can stay there if I like. But I tell them I won't need this piece of earth. I see my soul rise from the ground.

In spite of all the spiritual gifts I was receiving in my dreams, my body felt wretched. I could feel my mind teetering on the edge of the precipice.

I knew I had a choice. I could choose to remain in the world of Spirit. But a voice was telling me that my work was not done. I would have to return to ordinary life.

First I would have to visit the realm of the dead. I dreamed:

Marcela and I are at a ferry terminal. There are many people wait-ing to board. We have a small boat just for us, one that belonged to my father. People help us launch our boat, which I know how to pilot because my father taught me. Not my human father, but the heavenly Father.

I am preparing to cross the great water in my own craft, not with all the others taking the ferry. I am making my journey to the land of the dead but not with the dying. I am going with my shaman wife.

I had a new mission—to be a shaman. But wait! Hadn't I answered the call to be a shaman a long time ago? I'd even writ-ten a book about it: *Shaman, Healer, Sage.*

Now Spirit was offering me another lifetime within this one. I was being called to step into a new destiny, without self-importance, without the subtle seduction of worldly accomplishment. The externals of my life might not change, but my attitude had to.

I felt liberated. I was free. That night, I dreamed:

I am inside a breathing machine and friends are saying good-bye. I am unable to move or speak, but I am in bliss. They turn off life support. I have to pull myself out of the breathing apparatus to come back to life. I realize I can find eternity without dying. I rip the tube out of my mouth and breathe. I am alive.

I realized that I did not have to die. I could stay and heal myself so I could help others to heal. Once I made that choice, I felt my spirit extending roots into my body once again. Awe and wonder returned as my brain fog began to clear and I expe-rienced Oneness, where life and death flow seamlessly into each other and where I reside in infinity.

My good friend Mark Hyman, who wrote *Food: What the Heck Should I Eat?,* helped me put together a nutritional plan for healing my body. Mark and I co-lead seven-day detox programs for our clients in exotic locations. His plan for me included green juices in the morning and superfoods and supplements that detoxify the liver and brain.

Today, I'm fully recovered. More accurately, I'm *beyond* recovered. I'm a new person. My mind is functioning at a higher level than it has in decades. My brain is upgraded and so is my heart. And I have a new liver—not a transplant, but my own liver, fully regenerated. I was able to grow a new body.

Surgeons have long known that you can remove 80 percent of a person's liver, and it will grow back within two months. The liver's amazing ability to regenerate probably comes from being exposed to toxins back when our ancestors discovered which fruits and plants were edible through trial and error.

The liver isn't the only organ in the body that can regenerate itself. You grow a completely new heart every 15 years, your bones are only 2 years old, your lungs and skin are around 2 to 4 weeks old, and your intestines have changed all their cells within the last 3 days. With my own recovery, I began to understand that aging is what happens when your body loses its ability to regenerate itself, when healthy cells no longer replace sick and dying ones. Imagine what might happen if you could direct your body to grow only healthy, vibrant new cells.

The secret was in the healing plants from the Amazon. I found that the plants most treasured by shamans in the rain forest could help you to break in to the password-protected regions in your DNA where the instructions to grow a new body are stored. But the phytochemical properties alone were not enough; they simply opened the vault where the codes were kept. Their full power was unleashed only by the spiritual practices in this book.

In *Power Up Your Brain*, I wrote about the science of neuroplasticity and how you can trigger the production of neural stem cells that repair the brain with omega-3 fatty acids. During my health crisis, I learned that it's not just the brain that manufactures stem cells. Every organ in the body produces them, but we must learn how to turn on the genetic switches that will trigger repair and regeneration. Pluripotent stem cells will allow you to grow a new body that's healthier and more resilient. I call this system One

Spirit Medicine because it requires the power of Spirit for renewing the body. Diet, vitamins, supplements, and superfoods alone will not do it. It requires the experience of Oneness, the awareness of a reality where our separateness from creation and each other is an illusion—a trick of the mind. We truly are One.

As part of One Spirit Medicine, I offer the Grow a New Body program, which is backed by the latest breakthroughs in neuroscience. For the last decade, I've offered this program to clients who come to our weeklong retreats sponsored by The Four Winds Society. Participants leave with body and brain upgraded. Now, in this new edition of my book *One Spirit Medicine*, I offer you the same practices you would learn in these retreats, including the medicine plants and spiritual strategies that will help you return to health and keep your health for the rest of your life.

My health crisis was more extreme than most. But the fact is, we're all in a life-and-death struggle with the toxic forces of modern life that throw our health and well-being out of balance. With the knowledge in this book, you can get your "health span"—the length of time you're in optimal health—to equal your life span.

One of my clients had been diagnosed with advanced osteoporosis, and a year after completing the Grow a New Body program, her bone density had returned to what it was when she was in her 20s. Her condition is not uncommon. In the United States, 55 percent of persons over the age of 50 will develop osteoporosis. It is likely that these staggering statistics are due to the acidic Western diet, forcing our blood to use calcium to neutralize acid instead of building bone. And most medications designed to combat osteoporosis do not work, or have such terrible side effects as to make them downright dangerous. The latest science is showing that the supplements in my program, and others like it, can help you prevent osteoporosis and recover lost bone density. Dr. Roman Thaler and his fellow researchers at the Mayo Clinic have found that "the food-derived compound SFN (sulforaphane) epigenetically stimulates osteoblast activity and diminishes osteoclast bone resorption, shifting the balance of bone homeostasis and favoring bone acquisition and/or mitigation of bone resorption in vivo. Thus, SFN is a member of a new class of epigenetic compounds that could be considered for novel strategies to counteract osteoporosis."[1] Yes, you can even grow new bones in your body, and recover lost bone density! In Chapter 6, you will learn more about sulforaphane and other plant products that can do this.

Meanwhile, obesity, diabetes, attention deficit hyperactivity disorder (ADHD), and Alzheimer's disease are increasing at an alarming rate. One in three children born in America today will develop type 2 diabetes by the age of 15. Fifty percent of otherwise healthy 85-year-olds are at risk for Alzheimer's disease.[2] Alzheimer's is being called type 3 diabetes, linked to a gluten-rich, wheat-based diet and a stressed-out brain.[3]

The dreaded dementia and diabetes statistics are *not* inevitable, and we can escape that fate by making healthy lifestyle choices. Researchers in Finland studied 1,200 adults at risk for cognitive decline and discovered that those who maintained a diet of whole, unprocessed foods, including extra-virgin olive oil, fatty fish, and nutrient-dense fruits and vegetables, were not only able to maintain their brain health but improve it by 30 percent compared with controls.[4]

The Grow a New Body program I offer in my retreats and in this book can help you heal from the illnesses that are ravaging civilization today—but it can also do even more. The medicine men and women of old were masters of *prevention*. You do not have to be gravely ill to root out physical, emotional, and spiritual suffering and restore balance to your life. Using the program offered in these pages, you can feel better in a few days and begin to clear your mind and heal your brain in a week. And you will be well on your way to a new body that heals rapidly and ages gracefully, and a brain that supports you in forging a profound connection with Spirit and experiencing a renewed sense of purpose in life.

How to Use This Book

I've designed this book to guide you through the steps to grow the new body that will take you through the rest of your life. This requires that you upgrade your brain, so you can maintain a state of awareness I call Oneness. To get the most out of the process, I recommend reading the chapters in the order in which they're presented and trying the dietary practices and exercises before moving on in your reading.

Part I: Discovering Your Inner Healer introduces One Spirit Medicine; the invisible world of radiant, living energy that informs the visible world of the senses; and Spirit's role as the harmonizing force in your health. You'll be introduced to the tyrannical mind-set that has dominated humanity since the dawn of agriculture and understand how it drives us to war with ourselves and with each other, undermining our health and well-being.

Part II: Shedding the Old Ways identifies the myriad environmental and endogenous toxins (produced in the body) that we're exposed to and explains how to detoxify the body and the brain. You'll learn about the "second brain" in the digestive tract and how to upgrade the beneficial bacteria of your biome to eliminate toxins before they enter your blood or brain. You'll be introduced to superfoods that promote brain and gut repair, discover the toxic effects of grains and sugars, learn how our protein-rich diets are making you sick, and understand how ketosis helps you burn healthy fats and produce neural stem cells to repair and upgrade the brain.

In **Part III: Overcoming the Death That Stalks You**, you'll learn to transform dysfunctional emotional patterns founded on anger and fear, and how brain nutrients can help to improve higher-brain function and help you manage stress. You'll be introduced to the mitochondria, the power centers of your cells. Inherited from your mother, they represent the feminine life force. You'll learn how to reset the cells' "death clocks" and switch on longevity proteins controlled by mitochondria. You'll find out what free radicals and inflammation do to the body and how to reverse the damage. And you'll discover shamanic techniques that can upgrade your body and brain.

Part IV: From Stillness Comes Rebirth supports you in the process of letting go of old, unhealthy ways of thinking so that you can experience healing with One Spirit Medicine. You'll learn how to shed outworn narratives about your past and embrace a new, liberating personal story. You'll overcome fear of loss and change, and discover a new purpose for your life journey.

In **Part V: The Grow a New Body Program**, you'll put what you've learned into action. You'll dedicate seven days to this plan and repeat it every three months.

You will learn to change what and when you eat in order to enter into *ketosis* to activate the regions in the brain that will allow you to have an experience of Oneness. You will also learn to work with neuronutrients available at your health-food store that detoxify the body and brain and switch on the genes that create health and longevity. Lastly, you will learn how to do a soul retrieval to recover the vibrant and innocent parts of yourself that were lost because of childhood trauma.

PART I

DISCOVERING YOUR INNER HEALER

Chapter 1

MEDICINE
OF THE
SHAMANS

You are only a few days away from feeling well.

In the West we do not have a health-care system, we have a disease-care system that recognizes thousands of ailments and myriad remedies. One Spirit Medicine, on the other hand, identifies only one ailment and one cure. The ailment is alienation—from our emotions, from our bodies, from the earth, and from Spirit. The symptoms of this ailment are physical and emotional disease. The cure is the experience of Oneness, which restores inner harmony and facilitates recovery from all maladies, regardless of origin.

When our minds, our emotions, our relationships, or our bodies go out of kilter, we tend to ignore the problem until something goes very wrong—a scary diagnosis, a broken relationship, the death of a loved one, or simply an inability to function easily in everyday life. When things are a little bad, we read a self-help book or go to a workshop. When they're really bad, we bring in experts to fix the problem—oncologists to address cancer, neurologists to repair the brain, psychologists to help us find peace and understand our family of origin. But this fragmented approach to health is merely a stopgap. To truly heal, we need to rediscover the original recipe for wellness discovered millennia ago: One Spirit Medicine.

One Spirit Medicine states that the best way to heal and maintain health is to *grow a new body* on a regular basis. It recognizes the body as a *system,* not as a collection of parts that can be medicated or replaced when they go wrong. You cannot repair the heart without attending to the gut and the brain, and vice versa. And you can begin to grow a new body in as little as seven days. At the Center for Energy Medicine that I direct, every participant has found nearly 75 percent of all their symptoms alleviated within one week. You can do the same with the program in this book.

There are two food habits that will prevent you from growing a new body: excess sugar and excess protein. We've known about the evils of sugar and sugary drinks for some time. But new science confirms what our Paleolithic ancestors—who were gatherers and occasional, clumsy hunters—practiced: *periodic protein deprivation.* It turns out that excessive protein shuts down the longevity programs in our DNA. (But more on this later.)

We all want our health span to equal our life span. One Spirit Medicine can help you address the root cause of physical, mental, and emotional disease rather than just treating the symptoms. The words *health* and *healing* come from the Old English *haelen*, the root of *whole* and *holy.* As your brain begins to detox, your body will begin to repair and heal naturally, your relationships will cease to be emotional battlegrounds, and your sense of separation from nature and Spirit will dissolve.

At the heart of the Grow a New Body program is a new way of thinking about what you eat and when you eat it, using intermittent fasting, protein restriction, and fat for fuel to upgrade your brain. Then you will set up a carefully choreographed encounter in nature with the invisible world through a *vision quest*, which accelerates the body's self-repair and regeneration systems and reconnects you to your own deepest purpose. In indigenous cultures, it is customary to go into the wilderness to seek a vision. The early Christians would go into the desert and fast and pray. But the visionary epiphany can take place anywhere—even in your garden or a big city park.

Preparing the Brain

To grow a new body, we need to detoxify the brain and prime it for higher intelligence.

Mother Nature programs every species for longevity. She wants bees, butterflies, whales, and humanity to live a long time. But she does not care that individual bees, whales, or you and I have a long life. The way she does this is by programming the individual for reproduction. The more babies, the better the chances that the species will survive. She invests in the young and makes us fascinated with sex. It's amazing how quickly children heal from cuts and scrapes and broken bones, and how difficult it is for an older person to recover from an accident. The young fall in love, have babies, procreate. The young are the strongest, and the strongest survive.

Nature not only seeks the strongest but also the wisest. Intelligence trumps muscle and sinew and teeth. And she allows only two out of the millions of species on the earth to live into old age. In nearly every species, except orcas and humans, the female animal dies before menopause, when she is no longer useful for reproduction. Orcas and humans have some of the largest brains and greatest capacity for intelligence. Orca grandmothers mentor the youths, showing them coves they can hunt in and teaching them the ways of the sea. Human grandmothers traditionally had a role in guiding the young, one which has eroded in modern times.

Nature loves intelligence. The ancients called this wisdom *spirituality*. Not religion, which is a fixed set of beliefs and dogma about who your enemies are and how the world works.

Spirituality is about exploring the nature of the mind and the fabric of the cosmos through what the ancients called the experience of Oneness.

Later in the book, we will learn how spirituality requires that we activate regions in the brain that prefer to burn fats for fuel. We will learn that these regions are responsible for creativity, exploration, music, and science, and for hacking our biology to program us for longevity and health. The higher brain centers cannot function properly on glucose, the lower-grade fuel the body uses for everyday survival.

How Do We Do It?

Today's staccato, screen-dominated, I-want-it-now lifestyle keeps us in a constant state of stress. We need to be weaned off the stress hormones that promote a fight-or-flight mind-set and start producing the brain chemicals that create health, serenity, and joy. You cannot experience Oneness just by chanting *Om* or repeating a prayer. You need the brain chemistry that supports it. You can do this with the help of neuronutrients that enable the pineal gland to produce DMT, or dimethyltryptamine, a compound that has been referred to as the "spirit molecule."

DMT is found not just in the human brain but throughout nature: all plants, animals, and even trees produce it. DMT is the main component of ayahuasca, a psychedelic concoction brewed up by Amazon healers as an aid to visioning and psychic exploration. This bliss molecule provides the underlying brain chemistry for us to experience Oneness. The brain produces DMT when we dream, when we meditate, when we make love, and especially when we die. But the brain cannot produce the bliss molecules if it is flooded in stress molecules. We have to chill first, and change our diets.

To start, we must begin by switching to a diet rich in phytonutrients, or plant nutrients. *Phyto* comes from the Greek for plant, and phytonutrients account for the antioxidant, anti-inflammatory, and other amazing properties of certain plants.

The plants you will be using during the seven-day Grow a New Body program are loaded with epigenetic modifiers that switch on more than 500 genes that create health and switch off more than 200 genes that create disease. And you will be taking neuronutrients that support brain health.

Ridding yourself of toxins in your brain and body is essential to restoring physical and mental balance. You can't heal your emotions if your mind is careening unstoppably because your brain has been damaged by childhood trauma or pesticides in your food or mercury from your dental fillings. The supplements you will be taking in this program will help you eliminate years of toxins built up inside every cell in your body.

The final key is repairing your biome—the thousands of species of beneficial bacteria living in your mouth, skin, and gut. Upgrading your gut biome (also known as "flora") will help you upgrade your brain by allowing it to manufacture the neurotransmitters that you need to experience Oneness.

Preparing the Mind

To grow a new body, you don't need to shake a rattle or beat a drum as shamans of old did. What you *will* need to do is quiet your too-busy mind and return it to your natural, undomesticated self—to who you are without the trappings of roles and expectations, text messages, and to-do lists—the authentic *you* at your core. You will meet yourself in the quiet of your inner world during your vision quest and the practice of soul retrieval.

The shamanic exercises will help you shed outmoded stories about your past, limiting beliefs, and toxic behaviors, so you can begin to craft a new destiny infused with health and meaning. The practices will lead you to the experience of Oneness.

You Will Live to 100

The philanthropist Armand Hammer is credited with saying, "If I had known I was going to live this long, I would have taken better care of myself." Life expectancy for a 65-year-old American woman is nearly 85 years, and in Japan, it is 87 years. Man or woman, you should plan on living to the age of 100. But you don't want to spend that last 20 years of your life bedridden or unable to remember your grandchildren's names. You want to spend them in vibrant well-being, taking your humor, your vitality, your sexuality, and your good health into the last days of your life.

There is no question that the better educated are living longer. In a study published by the *Journal of the American Medical Association*, Raj Chetty and his co-authors found that the wealthiest 1 percent of American women live more than 10 years longer than the poorest 1 percent, and the gap between the wealthiest and poorest American men is almost 15 years.[1] How well you eat, how you exercise and look after yourself, and how much of your basic time and energy has to be dedicated to your family's survival affect your health and longevity. The better-educated Americans spend more than $30 billion a year in nutritional supplements.

Whatever your financial situation, you can improve your health span and life span with the Grow a New Body program. To do this, you'll eat a lot of vegetables—but also fats and some proteins, including fish, and fruit. The rain forest dwellers know the supernutrients I describe in this book that can turn on the dormant antioxidant mechanisms in every cell, quench free-radical activity in the brain, and switch on the longevity genes that prevent the illnesses associated with old age. And you do not need to be rich to do that, you just need to be smart.

As I've said, the eating style in the Grow a New Body program is based on the periodic protein deprivation of our ancestors. Numerous books have been written about the diet of our Paleolithic ancestors, many of which are misguided, but some are brilliant. (I am a particular fan of *Primal Fat Burner* by Nora Gedgaudas.) Few if any of these authors have lived with horticulturalists or studied modern-day hunter-gatherers—they have only read the research of others. In the years I spent in the Amazon, I discovered that the rain forest dwellers, who followed a similar eating style to our Paleolithic ancestors, were spared the diseases that ravage modern city dwellers. While yes, they eat meat, they don't do so every day, and certainly not in the form of bacon cheeseburgers! They would feast and then fast, depending on their luck foraging. Today we know that feasting and fasting is the key to regeneration and to growing a new body, and that we can detox and upgrade the brain to experience Oneness. (Also, just as important as diet is the stress-free lifestyle and the experience of Oneness with all life shared by these indigenous peoples.)

You don't need to look outside yourself to find health. You only have to look within. That's where you will receive One Spirit Medicine.

Chapter 2

SPIRIT AND THE INVISIBLE WORLD

*There is a sea of consciousness that is universal even though
we each perceive it from our own shore. It is a world that we
all share, one that can be experienced by every living being yet
is seldom seen by any. The shaman is the master of this
other world. He lives with one foot in the world of
matter and one foot in the world of Spirit.*

— From *Dance of the Four Winds*, by Alberto Villoldo
and Erik Jendresen

Years ago, I spent a summer in the Amazon rain forest, sponsored by a Swiss pharmaceutical giant that was hoping to find a bark or root that could become the next great cancer cure. After all, the jungle is nature's pharmacy, filled with exotic plants whose powers have yet to be discovered. I spent many months canoeing to villages that had seldom seen a white man, and wherever I went, I found there was no cancer, Alzheimer's, or heart disease, even among the elderly in the community. Clearly, the indigenous people of the area knew something about health that we Westerners didn't know. What was their secret?

I returned home with my backpack empty, to the annoyance of my sponsor, who couldn't believe I hadn't brought back the key ingredient for a blockbuster drug that would make us all rich and save lives at the same time. I did return, however, with something I thought more valuable—insights from the Amazon healers who had taken me under their wing. I learned that there were two magical ingredients to health. The first ingredient could be found only in the invisible matrix of the universe—what I call Oneness. The second ingredient was the plants that promote health, but do not treat specific disease. It took years of studying with indigenous healers before I began to comprehend how these work together.

Once you've experienced the invisible matrix of overlapping fields of consciousness, you recognize that the visible world of the senses, the physical world, is not the only reality. In fact, it's not even the dominant reality. The visible and invisible worlds are inextricably intertwined with almost mathematical precision, and once you've opened your eyes to this, you can dance between them.

The ancients knew all about these two worlds. In the Hindu Vedas, the invisible world is called *akasha*, or the vastness of space—the field of wisdom that forms the foundation of the cosmos. While Western science holds that the cosmos is made up of energy and matter, indigenous peoples consider the cosmos a living, intelligent field they know as Spirit.

The second ingredient comes from the world of plants—bushes, roots, and herbs that turn on the genes that create health and switch off the genes that create disease. Today we call these epigenetic modifiers, and science knows them as Nrf2 activators. You will learn how to use these supplements, and how they work, in a later chapter.

Vast and Omnipresent Spirit

Spirit is a vast and invisible field that we partner with to dream the world into being. It is not a deity with human whims, moods, jealousies, and temper tantrums like the Greek and

Roman gods displayed. Spirit does not ask you to sacrifice your firstborn child, or slay infidels, or destroy cities when their citizens have lost their way. Spirit is the creative matrix that keeps the cosmos evolving and renewing itself.

Spirit is always present in your life; you are an expression of its infinite potential, manifest in flesh and blood. And as you and Spirit are inseparable, you can experience the Oneness of all of creation within you. But our personal, individual awareness is merely a drop in the ocean of all consciousness. Unlike your mind, which thinks you're the center of the universe, your spirit is free of any obsession with *I.*

Awareness of our individuality, which we value so highly in our world, dissolves when we're in the expansive state of Oneness in the invisible world. And when the awareness of *I* returns, when we experience ourselves in the world, having returned to ordinary consciousness, our everyday problems somehow seem less burdensome.

When we engage with Spirit, we discover that Spirit responds with what we truly need, even if we do not fully comprehend the response at the time. And our relationship with Spirit is one of mutuality, so when Spirit calls, we have to be willing to answer the call, whether or not we understand what we're being asked to do and whether or not we want to do it. The biblical story of Jonah, who was swallowed by a whale when he refused God's call, teaches us that we want to be sure that we catch God on a whisper.

Years ago, when my children were little, I remember telling Spirit that I would respond to my calling when they were a bit older: I was using my children as an excuse to avoid my mission. But if you put off responding to Spirit until some future time—when you have enough money, or enough time, or enough sleep—then your contract with Spirit is likely to fall short of your wishes or expectations. This brings to mind a colleague at San Francisco State University where I was teaching. He had always wanted to play the cello, and he kept telling us all that when he retired he would dedicate himself to his music. Tragically, one week after he received his retirement, he passed away.

A Harmonizing Force

Most of us were taught that bad things happen because we have broken the rules established by a supernatural deity or somehow offended the gods. But Spirit is not a fickle deity who acts vindictively or tests our loyalty or seeks retribution if we make a mistake. In fact, Spirit is not a deity at all. Spirit is the great balancing force of life itself. It brings harmony, not punishment.

Misfortune and disease is simply an imbalance in the natural harmony. It occurs when we're alienated from the wisdom of the invisible world, when we're trapped in limiting and disempowering stories about our lives. When all we see is the material world, our survival instincts kick into gear. We mistakenly believe that the only way to avoid illness, conflict, or suffering is by fighting for survival and exerting power over others. But in fact, our greedy, selfish, manipulative actions lead to the very illness, conflict, and suffering we're trying so hard to avoid.

That's not to say that we are the authors of all of the misfortune that befalls us. Sometimes what we're experiencing are the consequences of an imbalance we personally had no part in creating. The Ebola virus is an example. This deadly virus was once contained within a 10-square-mile forest in Africa, but when the forest was cut down for lumber, the virus lost its natural habitat and quickly spread to animals and humans in the surrounding area. Many of the people who have died from Ebola had nothing to do with cutting down the forest, but they suffered mightily from it nonetheless.

Most microbes only harm you when your body is out of balance and your immune system isn't responding properly. Eighty-five percent of your immune system is in your gut, regulated by your gut flora. You may not have the power to ensure that no deadly parasite will attack you, but you do have the power to prevent and correct imbalances in your gut. If you're living in imbalance, you're in a state of separation from Spirit. To dream a healthier, happier life into being, you need to correct your relationship to Spirit. But first you need to repair your gut. (More on this in Chapter 4.)

The Veil between the Two Worlds

In our quest for the scientific exploration of the universe, we have forgotten about personal exploration of the invisible realm of the mind and what we can find there. In the West we use our mind to study nature, to explore mathematics, but we have neglected to use the mind to study the mind. When you turn the mind within to study itself, you find peace and freedom from the suffering that exists in the material world. You find the wisdom that infuses all creation. Much like the microscope is the instrument to study the very small, the mind is the instrument to study the invisible world. But if the invisible world is so marvelous, why aren't we spending all our time there?

The sages say that the reason we are born into a body in the physical world is to evolve and grow, to acquire maturity and wisdom. To use a metaphor from physics, when we're embodied, we're like a photon in a particle state; while in the invisible world, we're like a photon in a field state. The particle state is our "local" nature—flesh and blood, sitting on a couch reading. The field state is our "nonlocal" nature, in which we extend to the farthest reaches of the universe and are at one with all things. When we die and leave this body behind, we return to our nonlocal nature, to our field state, to invisible Oneness. But the sages of old learned to experience their field without dying—to taste Oneness while still in the world.

Our field state, the one we inhabit in between births, encompasses all of creation. The field is insubstantial: we don't have enough substance to contain our awareness. The ancient Maya called the consciousness needed to experience this state of Oneness the "jaguar body." The jaguar-shamans were individuals who had defeated death and developed awareness of their infinite field state, and they brought this wisdom back to their kings. This is why the jaguar is such a powerful symbol throughout the Americas; the feline represents the journey beyond death, exploring the state of omniscience in the field, and returning to the embodied state of the living. After acquiring the jaguar wisdom, we understand that there never was a locked gate between us and the invisible world. The invisible world exists alongside the visible one, ever present and accessible. We can bring its wisdom into our world at any time to provide healing and balance.

The way we do this is by activating the circuitry in the brain that allows us to experience our interconnectedness to all things and all beings in the cosmos. These higher-order neural networks, like all neural networks, are made up of brain cells connected to each other, of neurons that fire together and wire together. They are in a region of the brain known as the neocortex, or "new brain," which thrives on bliss and the experience of Oneness, while other parts of the brain are more concerned with survival and separation of friend from foe. This more recently evolved part of the brain has a favorite food source: ketone bodies, or fats, which are like jet fuel for the brain. You cannot explore the invisible world of Spirit with your predatory and more primitive limbic brain, which feeds primarily on sugars and is terrified of death, ghosts, and shadows lurking in the night.

Today the interface between our senses and our machines is moving us ever closer to being able to access all the knowledge in the world instantaneously. But this is not the kind of omniscient awareness I'm referring to. The awareness I speak of is the mind's ability, in the field state, to experience the cosmos firsthand, across the farthest reaches of space and beyond time. This is the magic potion that I discovered in the Amazon, the medicine that heals the longings of the soul and helps us deal with the stressors of life. With this potion we can become the architects of a destiny infused with health and long life.

The thick doorway between us and the invisible matrix is regulated by the sugars in our diet, by the excess protein in our food, and by the toxins in our brain. If we change our diet, repair our broken brains, and learn to use fats for fuel, we can break down the gate that keeps us from the Oneness that is obvious from the perspective of our higher brain.

When the conquistadors first arrived to the Americas, the indigenous people on the coast of Mexico didn't perceive their wooden ships. Their scouts saw only the billowing white sails. The Indians weren't blind or foolish or crazy. Having no concept of such large boats, their minds simply erased what their eyes registered. Research shows that our mental biases are so strong that we easily dismiss sensory information that doesn't fit with our preconceived notions about reality. A century and a half ago, doctors scoffed at the notion of viruses and bacteria that caused infectious diseases. After all, they couldn't see the alleged "bugs," so how could the bugs be real? We fail to grasp what's right in front of us. Our mind dismisses the information.

Luminous Energy Field

How does the invisible world of Spirit impact health and healing? Surrounding the physical body is a luminous energy field, or LEF, that informs our cells and biome—the community of microorganisms in and on our body—about how to live in harmony. The LEF is invisible, though there are people who perceive this energy as an aura, a halo of color around a person's body. With practice, you can sense this energy. (Try it now: rub your palms together briskly for a few seconds, then slowly separate your hands slightly and try to feel heat or a kind of "static" in the air between your palms.)

The LEF can be thought of as the software that instructs your DNA, the hardware, to repair your body. It does this through your brain and nervous system, and the chakras or energy centers in the body. You can upgrade the quality of your LEF through meditation, walks in nature, and prayer. But if you do not update your LEF, or if your brain is full of toxins, and your field cannot upgrade your body, then you simply create your health according to default programs inherited from your family. You replicate the physical maladies and the psychological stories and dramas that your ancestors lived with and died from.

Despite our longing to see ourselves as different, better, and more enlightened than our parents, we tend to perpetuate their health challenges and emotional issues, repeating them in our own lives in one form or another. Unless we upgrade our LEF through the experience of Oneness, we will live the way they lived and die the way they died. Our bodies start to develop cancer cells that forget to die and want to live forever, and our systems for keeping them in check will not be able to sustain the battle.

Today we know that 90 percent of the human body consists of bacteria that are not us. Only 10 percent of our body is made up of our own DNA, and the rest belongs to our biome. So does this mean that "I" am only that 10 percent? No. I am the energy field that organizes this amazing living colony that has a sense of self, of I-ness. The 100 trillion cells of my colony are kept humming in harmony, operating through my brain and nervous system. Nature made us this way, no doubt figuring that it was better to have one brain coordinating it all than to give each cell its own mind and the freedom to decide what is best for the whole colony. Rather than freedom, that would be a free-for-all.

Your LEF is a biomagnetic field, which does not end where your skin ends but rather extends to the farthest reaches of the universe, diminishing in intensity, yet never vanishing altogether. Your LEF contains stars and galaxies within it.

If you have heard the expression that thoughts become things, well, this is how it happens. Your LEF will organize the physical reality around you to mirror your thoughts and beliefs faithfully. If you don't upgrade the wisdom in your LEF and choose instead to stay stuck in the same old thoughts—*Mom ruined my life,* or *The stork dropped me off at the wrong home,* or *Heart disease runs in my family,* or whatever old story you habitually run—you create this in your life.

In Eastern philosophy, this cause-and-effect is known as karma. And being stuck in karma is not a fun way to go through life. You do not want to live as the effect of an earlier cause, whether of the genetics that run in your family or of your early life trauma—unless, of course, you want to spend a good part of your life in therapy! When you raise the quality of your LEF, you can begin to express the genes for health and longevity, and live a more original and rewarding life. To do this you begin by detoxifying your brain and feeding it the neuronutrients and fuel that will give you access to the experience of Oneness where you can upgrade your field, what I call downloading version 7.0 of the human software.

It's much harder for us to raise the quality of our LEF today than it was 100 years ago, or 10,000 years ago, when our Paleolithic ancestors lived in graceful communion with nature. The toxins in our body and nervous system from pesticides, man-made chemicals, mercury that has been extracted from the earth, and other poisons did not exist a century ago. We no longer readily experience unity with all creation except for brief moments. No matter how arduously we meditate, the invisible matrix of Spirit seems to elude us.

But it doesn't have to.

Our LEF is a gateway to the invisible matrix of wisdom where everything is intertwined, where every thought we have impacts every cell in our body and every molecule in the cosmos. Quantum physics offers us an apt metaphor in the phenomenon known as entanglement: two particles can be mysteriously interlinked in such a way that even if they are at opposite ends of the galaxy, if you change the direction in which one particle is spinning, the other immediately reverses its spin. At first scientists thought entanglement might be a demonstration of faster-than-light communication. Later they understood that it was simply the nature of related particles. The sages of the Amazon and Andes that I studied with believe that entanglement is the nature of all of creation, that we are all related. That is why they—and many Native Americans—refer to all living beings as "all my relations."

When you participate in the shared awareness of all Creation, you recognize your Oneness with all beings and with nature. How can you harm the earth or other beings when you and they are inseparable? Conversely, how can you not attend to your own healing if you care about your fellow beings? Once you've awakened to Oneness, the idea of looking out for yourself at the expense of others is inconceivable.

It's not practical or easy to work your way through a to-do list when you're in a state of Oneness. But once you experience your interconnectedness with the cosmos, what you put on your to-do list is likely to change, and your ability to complete the list without sabotaging yourself will almost certainly improve.

Awakening Your Invisible Self

When we sleep, we are awake in our dreams. When we are awake, we are sound asleep in the field where dreams happen. Dreams, meditation, deep contemplative study, music, and prayer are common ways of learning about the invisible realm. But these experiences are often fleeting, vanishing as we make our way from the bed to the coffee maker. When we dream, we are in a timeless world, one minute encountering our long-deceased relatives, the next traversing some fantastic landscape. But when we awaken, no matter how vivid the images, they often slip from awareness. In the West, psychologists trained in dream analysis are just about the only people who understand the importance of the dream life. Yet the Amazon peoples I studied with would share dreams every morning, looking to them for answers to pressing questions or wisdom to be passed on to the village.

Have you noticed that in your dreams you never seem to have a physical body, never seem to bump into tables or chairs? In dreams we are pure awareness. In the invisible world we are formless and self-less, within an expanse that is infinite and blissful. We are our LEF. It is only in the visible world that we bump into tables, fall off cliffs, encounter suffering and disease, and of course where we learn and grow the most. To the indigenous peoples I studied, embodied life isn't the only and ultimate reality: the invisible realm of spirit is the primary reality, and the luminous self is the enduring self.

As you grow a new body, you will also grow your recognition of your nature as both a spiritual being and a physical being, a field and a particle. It's inevitable. Newly aware of a self that is undying, you can live fearlessly.

This awareness will exorcise the fear of death from every

cell in your body. Your higher brain will allow you to understand that there is only life after life, that death is simply a brief change in status from a visible to an invisible existence.

And the discovery of your ageless-timeless self will allow you to grow a new body that heals, ages, and dies differently.

Chapter 3

DETHRONING
THE TYRANT KING

Know that the mind is mad.

In museums and at amusement parks, children are drawn to models of the fiercest of the dinosaurs, *Tyrannosaurus rex*, or *T. rex*. The *Spinosaurus* and *Giganotosaurus* may have been bigger carnivores, and *Diplodocus* and *Apatosaurus* were many times the size of *T. rex*, but he had the good fortune to have his brand established first—at the turn of the 20th century, Victorian crowds eagerly bought tickets to view the skeleton of this beast. The fearsome dinosaur was given a name worthy of sending shivers down the spine of an eight-year-old and assigned a reputation that fulfills a mythological purpose: he represents the tyrannical king who will destroy us if we don't bow to his power. Although we now know the *Tyrannosaurus rex* probably had feathers, in our imagination he had a thick, impenetrable hide that made him an undefeatable predator.

The myth of the ferocious ruler also lives on in the large-cat house at the zoo. The sharp teeth and bold mane of the male lion impress onlookers as he yawns behind the glass. Even though we now know it's the smaller, sleeker female lion who does the hunting while her male partner looks on, the peering crowds ignore the informational card at the side of the exhibit and gaze in awe at the "king of the jungle."

T. rex and the male lion seem powerful because the image of a formidable creature ruling over us is deeply rooted in the human psyche. The notion of a warrior-ruler has been internalized to the point that we think of the rational mind as the dominant force of our being, lording over our thoughts, feelings, body, and spirit. We're told from infancy that our large, complex brains are what separate us from the rest of the animal kingdom. The everyday mind truly believes that it's in charge, running our thoughts and emotions, not to mention our lives. We believe that to change our habits, our addictions, our relationships, and our feelings, all we have to do is change our mind. And so we keep changing our mind—without fixing our relationships, improving our health, or healing our emotions.

The truth is that we cannot really change our minds without changing our brains. And while the mind is not located in the brain, it operates through the brain and nervous system. After you detox your brain and begin to manufacture your brain's natural bliss molecule (DMT), you will be able to transform toxic relationships, upgrade your health, and repair your emotions more easily. Then you will discover that the ordinary mind is not the ultimate tool for creating health, abundance, love, and well-being. That's not to say we can't enlist the mind to help us heal. The mind-body connection has long been acknowledged as a factor in wellness as well as illness. The mind I'm referring to is the domineering limbic brain, which believes it's in charge and in control, and that lives in scarcity, anger, and fear. This is the brain that guided our Neanderthal cousins and that rebels when things don't turn out the way we want them to, and that wants to be the captain of the ship.

You will discover a more effective tool: a relationship with Spirit and the invisible world. But to do this you need to bring on-line the higher brain that can have a spiritual experience. You cannot control a spiritual experience, you have to surrender to it. This requires a higher mind that we attain when we begin burning fats for fuel, and combusting a ketone known as β-hydroxybutyrate. Otherwise you will be like the Aztec scouts that missed the great wooden ships of the Europeans because such massive crafts were not in their ordinary reality.

The Lord of the Dawn

During my early work in anthropology, when I visited cultures that lived much like their Paleolithic forebears, I was surprised to find how present the sacred was in their lives. Many of their legends speak about a heavenly being who walked the earth bringing wisdom. He was known as Quetzalcoatl, the feathered serpent, Lord of the Dawn to the Aztec and Hopi.

Quetzalcoatl was the ever-returning God, associated with Venus, the morning star. The legends say that he returns in every new era to bring renewal and wisdom, and he represents our own eternal return to the earth, lifetime after lifetime. His legacy is to continually renew the fertile soil, to replenish your body, your thinking, and your village. Quetzalcoatl teaches that mortal existence is brief and we have to cherish it and protect it, as it is extremely difficult to earn a physical body. You wanted long life and good health so you could learn the lessons you came to learn in this world. The shamans discovered the edible greens that are rich in phytonutrients and that ensured good health during our all-too-brief lives.

What an extraordinary collaboration there is between human beings and the plant kingdom. We are perfect symbionts: oxygen, the waste product of plant respiration, sustains life for humans, and our respiratory waste, carbon dioxide, sustains life for the plants. Plants turn sunlight into nutrient-dense foods we can use. For our ancestors, survival in the wilderness was a natural outcome of respectful interaction with nature. Knowing which berries were nutritious and which were poisonous and where to find edible roots required humans to communicate with green life in a way incredible to most of us today.

Indigenous people who are carrying on the tradition of respectful dialogue with nature will tell you that they know the qualities of plants not through trial and error but because the plants speak to them. The shamans discovered a category of plants that did not treat disease, but that created health.

During my journeys in the Amazon, I noticed that there were two distinct categories of plant medicine. The first were remedies for specific ailments. If you had a headache or a fever from malaria, for example, you would go to what I call the "aspirin tree"—a white willow or a cinchona—and prepare a remedy from the bark. This is the kind of medicine that we practice in the West: we find a remedy to treat the symptom.

The other category of plants creates health. They help you to grow a new body by turning on the longevity genes inside every cell, by detoxifying the brain, and by switching on the natural production of pluripotent stem cells. They work by upregulating Nrf2, the body's master regulator of aging and detoxification, to create health. In the Amazon these plants include cat's-claw and a dozen species of *shihuahuaco*. Like the Chinese sages who have been using ginseng for more than 2,000 years, the shamans benefited from the neuroprotective properties, the ability to switch on the production of neural stem cells, the power to switch on the longevity genes (SIRT-1 genes), and to detoxify the brain.[1]

We find similar properties in the cruciferous vegetables, including broccoli and Brussels sprouts, and spices like turmeric and black pepper. They are rich in phytonutrients that detoxify and upgrade the brain. This type of plant medicine helps us switch on the circuitry that overrides the tyrannical mind. We'll explore these superfoods in detail in Chapter 6, as they are essential for growing a new body.

So how did we lose this intimate connection with Spirit and the natural world? When did we stop speaking with the rivers and the trees? Anthropologist Jared Diamond traces it back 10,000 years to the agricultural revolution, when humans exchanged the Paleolithic hunter-gatherer diet for a diet based on agricultural grains. Diamond calls this dietary shift "the worst mistake in the history of the human race."[2] It led to centuries of war and conflict, he says, and gave rise to society after society of cruel masters, ruthless warriors, and hapless slaves.

With a diet based on wheat, barley, rice, and maize—grains with a high glycemic index, or blood-glucose elevating potential—our farming ancestors were essentially living on sugar. Our bodies and brains are still suffering the health consequences of this dietary shift. A brain steeped in sugar is sluggish and dull. In Chapter 4, you'll discover more about grains and how toxic they are to the digestive system and brain, and about the harmful effects of gluten, the proteins in cereal grains.

The rise of agriculture brought with it the notion that survival and security depended on a powerful divine-king who could rally forces to protect the land, the peasants, and the grain stores. Humans became fearful and warlike. Direct experience of the divine gave way to religions overseen by intermediaries and power brokers between God and man.

We need to bring our connection to Spirit and natural forces back into the healing equation. To find peace within ourselves and live harmoniously with all beings on the planet, we need to shift our allegiance away from the tyrannical, sugar-fueled, grain-fed mind-set. We must go back to the primarily plant-based diet of our ancient ancestors and their way of experiencing the Oneness of the cosmos.

To achieve this, we need to upgrade our neural circuitry.

The Limbic Brain and Neural Networks for Fear

When the mind is behaving tyrannically, it's running ancient programs belonging to the limbic brain that focus on survival, and the primary emotion is fear. When we're in its grip, we see danger everywhere. The programs of the limbic brain are known as the Four Fs—feeding, fighting, fear, and fornicating. The limbic brain craves sweet comfort foods when you are feeling sad or insecure. Feed it sugar and this brain keeps operating at a dull level of awareness that does not lead to an experience of Oneness.

This brain helped us to survive the Ice Age and is obsessed with having food and sex; it craves mind-dulling alcohol and drugs, and is biased toward aggression, emotional withdrawal, and self-preservation. When we cut off its supply of sugars, its instincts can be overridden by the neocortex, the "new" brain, which allows us to learn, create, and envision new futures. The neocortex is programmed for beauty, whether it's found in a Mozart concerto or an elegant mathematical solution. The new brain needs ketones to override the programs of the more ancient limbic brain. On a carbohydrate diet, it sputters along, coughing up the occasional creative revelation but no lasting insights.

The limbic brain, driven by pleasure seeking and emotional drama, does not thrive on spiritual experiences. It settles for religions that turn its biases and prejudices into divine commandments that address its basic survival needs. It does not long for an elegant dance with Oneness.

The limbic brain evolved while we were sitting quietly by the river's edge or watching the sun set lazily over the African savannah, and is not geared to the rhythm of the digital world. Under stress, primitive emotion overtakes us, and we become blind with jealousy or rage, paralyzed with fear, or so riddled with anxiety that we can't think straight. When it becomes overstimulated, it hijacks the entire neural apparatus, restricting blood flow to the frontal lobes of the brain, so we can no longer come up with creative solutions to problems.

Often we're not even aware that we're operating out of instinctual fear—we think the world is a dangerous place, that there are tigers or viruses around the corner waiting to eat us, that there aren't enough resources to go around, and that death means the end of our existence. Beliefs like these become etched into the neural networks in the limbic brain. Each time we think dark or fearful thoughts, we reinforce these networks.

Neural networks are information superhighways that quickly interpret what we perceive through the senses. They tell us red means danger, green means go, who is sexy, who is dull. They hold a dynamic map of our world and how our reality works. This map contains sights, sounds, scents, memories, and early childhood experiences. Many of our maps of reality are formed in the womb, as the mother's stress hormones pass through the placental barrier to the fetus. So if your mother was not sure she could count on her partner to protect her and her baby, your reality will be one in which you can't count on people to be there for you, or where the world will not support your endeavors. If, on the other hand, your mother was confident she could count on her beloved and her family and community, your map will reveal a world you can count on—and will infuse this reality into your relationships.

These neural networks become stronger as your day-to-day experience proves your map true, with more connections between neurons formed every time that pathway is used. Over the years, this path becomes the road most traveled and eventually the only route used. A brain scan will actually show neural networks in a particular area of the brain "lighting up" as you think certain thoughts. The opposite is true as well: when a neural network falls into disuse, the void in that area of the brain will show up on a scan. So even if you have a spiritual awakening during a weekend meditation retreat, unless you make a conscious effort to reinforce that insight once you return to your everyday existence, the epiphany will fade away.

Our neural networks make us creatures of habit. We stop having innovative thoughts and original ideas very early on. In fact, most of our neural networks are set by an early age, when we stop imagining houses in the clouds. And traumatic childhood experiences make us less resilient and creative, affirming negative beliefs about reality and strengthening the neural superhighways in the limbic brain that confirm this. And early life traumas correlate with higher levels of alcoholism, heart disease, depression, teen pregnancy, and many negative behaviors that in turn reshape our brains.[3]

The childhood fears, the anger, the suffering, and the feelings of abandonment encoded in our neural networks cause us to repeat the underlying themes of these memories, even if we don't recall the events themselves. As I reflect back on my own life, I notice that I have always suffered around the same themes—lost love, hurt, and abandonment. And fear. When I moved to New York City for a summer, decades ago, I arrived at my new apartment on a hot and muggy day. A bunch of beefy guys in sweaty T-shirts were sitting on the front steps. I was convinced I'd moved into a neighborhood of muggers and killers. Later, I discovered these men were my neighbors, came to know them, and found they couldn't have been nicer. I had unknowingly superimposed fear-filled childhood memories on these innocent neighbors.

Psychological themes run in families, passed down from parent to child. In the Amazon, they call this a generational curse. It can trigger heart disease or cancer. Autoimmune diseases, which involve the immune system attacking its own cells, often run in families with poor emotional boundaries—family members have trouble acknowledging what is yours and what is mine.

Whatever willpower we exert to change our habits, we often fall back into the old themes because of our ever-efficient neural networks. The good news is that we can rewire our neural networks for joy and more nourishing outcomes. But first we have to detoxify the brain. Remember, the poisons in our food and water are stored in fat cells, and the brain is largely made of fat. We cannot lay neural networks for bliss, creativity, or curiosity if our brain cells are loaded with toxins.

Neuroplasticity

Neuroplasticity, the mechanism by which our experiences affect the brain's functioning and structure, is a relatively new discovery for science. However, this cutting-edge discovery also matches what sages have known for millennia about how the world molds and shapes the brain. Not so long ago we believed that after the brain developed during childhood, it remained unchanged for the rest of our lives. Today we know that in response to an injury, or as a result of an epiphany or personal realization, individual neurons can change and even large-scale transformation of the brain, known as cortical remapping, can occur.

Neural networks act like filters that screen out certain experiences, allowing us to perceive only a limited slice of reality. So like the old Aztec scouts, we will fail to notice the conquistadors' ships, which later seem so obvious to us. We may fail to read the emotional warning signs from the person we are dating, before we become entangled in a toxic relationship.

Your neural networks create self-fulfilling prophecies. If you believe the world is full of thieves and liars, then that is what you will encounter. Talk therapy isn't very effective in dismantling the neural networks formed during childhood trauma. Too often, instead of helping us write a better story, it only reinforces the old script.

Studies show that the brain can remap itself very quickly, that in effect you can teach an old dog new tricks. In a 2005 study, medical students' brains were imaged using a brain-scan device before and after their exams. In a few months, the gray matter in the young doctors' brains increased significantly, indicating that the learning was clearly forming new neural networks in their brains and increasing their brain volume.[4] Since 2000, scientists have discovered that neurogenesis—the birth of new brain cells—happens *regularly*, particularly in the hippocampus, the brain structure associated with learning and memory. The shamans discovered the plants that triggered the production of neural stem cells without being able to explain the science.

Tasting Oneness from the fractured world of the limbic brain can help you change lanes in the information superhighway in your head so that you see the world with new eyes. It becomes easier to shed old stories and write new, more interesting, and more beneficial ones that will guide you to live in abundance and fearlessly.

Today we know the science—and we start by ridding our brain of toxins that prevent us from experiencing Oneness.

PART II

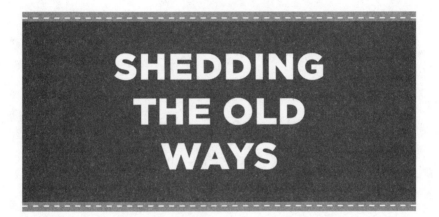

SHEDDING
THE OLD
WAYS

Chapter 4

DETOXIFYING THE GUT-BRAIN

I listen to my stomach and force myself to meditate on its groans. I imagine I can see the walls of my stomach rubbing against each other, muscles straining, and each contraction brings up a forgotten image from my childhood: mother, father, beach, happy. Father gone. Scared. Alone. Adolescence, love, lies, conceit, and deceit are all rolled into one. Whom do I pray to for forgiveness when I no longer believe in anything?

Hiram Bingham was the discoverer of Machu Picchu, and I have chosen to retrace his footsteps through the jungles of Peru to the mythic Inca City of Light. It's curious that when a "civilized" man is shown a place where natives have lived for centuries, he is called its discoverer— as if the natives had been keeping it a secret from the rest of the world.

Now I am camping at a cave just below the deserted ruins. Fasting for three days before I enter the citadel. Otherwise, the shamans tell me, I will miss the "spiritual" Machu Picchu. All I would see would be a pile of stone, not the invisible city that overlies the ruins. Will I be able to see through the mist, part the veils of this ancient palace?

And why do I have to do it on an empty stomach? The old man said, "So you can meet the beast within you and leave it outside the ruins." The beast turns out to be my entire past: the search for glory disguised as adventure, the ego rewards of revealing the treasures of ancient cultures to the world. The beast is me.

All the loose ends, all the polluted relationships, all the sorrows and joys—amazing what rises to the surface when you stop eating three meals a day, even for just a couple of days. I know that despite my lean frame, I have enough body fat to live off for months. But hunger is a great teacher. No wonder the psychology of the West is oral and anal.

— FROM *DANCE OF THE FOUR WINDS*, BY ALBERTO VILLOLDO
AND ERIK JENDRESEN

You have a second brain in your gut, and it's every bit as important as the brain in your head. This second brain is a network of more than 100 million neurons that communicate directly with the brain in your skull. Its neurons form a lattice-like sheath surrounding your entire digestive tract, a nearly 30-foot-long tube that runs from your mouth to your anus. This "gut brain" isn't concerned with poetry, love, philosophy, or whether there's life after death. Its work is the daily grind of digestion: breaking down food to extract the nutrients, absorbing those nutrients, and then eliminating waste. The gut communicates with your brain through the vagus nerve, which snakes up through the body from the gut, tells your brain how hungry or satisfied you are, and relays the messages of your gut-instinct.

The gut produces 90 percent of the serotonin in the body. Serotonin is both a hormone and a neurotransmitter and plays a crucial role in developing our forebrain, the region of the neocortex where learning, spirituality, and the higher emotions such as love or altruism can be experienced. Serotonin also enhances the growth of neurons in the region in the brain that enables us to have new experiences (the hippocampus). When this part of the brain is damaged by the stress hormones cortisol and adrenaline, we no longer learn anything new. We live in a world of "been there, done that," unable to have a new experience, an epiphany, a discovery, or to fall in love again. Have you seen an older couple walking in the park, holding hands tenderly? You need serotonin to stay in love, to wake up to the same person every morning and discover something new about them.

At dusk, with the changing light, our pineal gland converts serotonin into melatonin to signal the brain that it's time to release the ordinary world and enter the realm of sleep and dreams. Serotonin is probably the most ancient and universal hormone in the evolution of life; it's found in plants, animals, fungi, and even bacteria. Some call it the "feel good" or "happiness" hormone. It is chemically analogous to DMT, the "spirit molecule," described earlier. However, if the flora in your gut has been damaged, it won't produce serotonin and you'll be unable to manufacture the bliss molecules or enjoy the poetry of Rumi.

Today, DMT is a doorway used by many seekers in the Western world to venture into spiritual territory that was once the exclusive domain of shamans and native psychonauts. "DMT can . . . really open up the layers of your ego," explains Mitch Schultz, director of the documentary *DMT: The Spirit Molecule,* about psychiatrist Rick Strassman's pioneering research on DMT and spiritual experience. "Pulling back those layers of the ego, you start to get a sense of that perfect awareness of your being. And to me that is more real than real, if you will. More real than this hallucination that we're living in on a daily basis."

The pineal gland does not produce enough DMT for us to "see" musical notes or have a psychedelic trip. But it manufactures enough for us to have the experience of Oneness, and a sense of our interconnectedness with all creation. You need abundant serotonin to meditate, to make love, and to forgive yourself and others. Attending to the health of your gut-brain, where your serotonin is manufactured, will help you achieve this. Supplementing tryptophan, an essential amino acid, will help you to boost serotonin levels, balance your mood, sleep better, and support the production of DMT.

Western Medicine Ignores the Gut

Western medicine is using its best efforts to limit the ravages caused by our poor eating habits and sedentary lifestyles. According to the Kaiser Family Foundation, 90 percent of Americans over 65 rely on at least one prescription drug to treat an ailment.[1] We have thousands of medications to address symptoms but almost none to address the underlying causes of the imbalances that lead to disease.

Many of the diseases of modern living begin in the gut, and disturbances in the colony of microorganisms in the gut affect the functioning of the brain. When the biome becomes unbalanced with harmful microorganisms, they begin to produce toxins that wreak havoc with your immune system and alter your mood. If the bugs in your belly are not happy, you are not happy, no matter how many self-help books you read or what kind of yoga you do.

Lining your gut are 10 to 12 layers of good bacteria that are in charge of turning fish, broccoli, or scrambled eggs into *you*, and producing all the vitamins that you need. Each layer is populated by different species, and after the first layer of bacteria eat, they "poop"—and this is what the next layer feeds on. Each layer eats what the layer above it rejects until the very last layer "poops" the amino acids, vitamins, and minerals our bodies need to grow and repair. We are the very bottom rung of the food chain!

Think about that the next time you reach for a blueberry muffin or a sugar-rich protein bar. Are the bugs in your gut going to enjoy that meal, or are they going to be unhappy because what they really love are the fiber-rich vegetables, fats, and proteins that they can convert into the amino acids we require?

Although antibiotics do kill undesirable parasites in our body, they also indiscriminately kill the good bacteria we *want* in our biome. This attack on our flora wreaks havoc in our gut. A full course of antibiotics can destroy five or six of the layers in the bacterial sandwich in your gastrointestinal (GI) tract, so that you can be eating the very healthiest organic food but not be absorbing any of its nutrients because the good bacteria that do the heavy breaking down of foods are not present. Meanwhile, bad bugs are developing resistance to our best antibiotics, forcing doctors to turn to increasingly more powerful medications to combat them, which create even more damage to our sensitive flora. Many companies sell probiotics, good bacteria meant to replenish your gut biome; however, you'll soon learn why ingesting them is seldom effective.

Even if you haven't taken antibiotics in a while, they may be affecting your gut biome through unexpected sources! Did you know that 75 percent of all antibiotics sold in the U.S. are sold to ranchers to use on their livestock, which then end up on our dinner plate—and then in *us*? Just be sure you buy antibiotic-free, organic, free-range meats.

The bugs in our gut are intelligent, in the same way that a colony of bees or an anthill is intelligent. Our flora want to protect the health of the colony and do not like parasites any more than we do. When the colony is healthy, it will protect you from invading parasites and viruses. If your gut flora is damaged, it takes only 10 Salmonella bacteria to produce a gastrointestinal infection that will have you repeatedly running to the bathroom, with a high fever to boot. But if your flora is strong, it takes more than 1,000,000 of the same bacteria to produce a gastrointestinal infection.[2]

In the West, if you're suffering from anxiety, brain fog, or depression, most physicians or psychologists aren't going to pay attention to the balance between beneficial and non-beneficial flora in your gut. It's unlikely that your gastroenterologist will ask about your mental and emotional stress. I recently took my mother to the doctor, and the first thing he asked her was, "What medications are you taking?" That same day, I took my dog to the veterinarian, and the first thing she asked was, "What do you feed your dog?" I decided that if I got sick again, I would make an appointment to go see my vet first!

We know that our thoughts, beliefs, and feelings influence the physical structure of the brain. And we know that the gut regulates our mood, and gut imbalances can lead to depression and anxiety. Once you've upgraded your gut with the super-probiotics I suggest in Chapter 6, you will find it easier to make changes in your habits and relationships.

Ask yourself the following:

- *Do you sleep well?*
- *Can you recall your dreams in the morning when you wake up?*
- *Are you able to dream lucidly, knowing you're dreaming while you're in the dream?*
- *Do you learn rapidly?*
- *Are you able to adapt to new situations easily?*
- *Are you able to leave work stress in the office and not take it home?*

If you answered no to any of these questions, you need to upgrade your gut.

Toxins That Degrade Brain Function

Our guts contain over 1,000 varieties of good microbes—including what one researcher calls "a virtual zoo of bacteria"—outnumbering by ten to one the cells that are strictly us. Like I said, the colonies of microbes in our skin, mouth, and gut don't like parasites, and they particularly do not like big predatory yeast like *Candida albicans*, an opportunistic pathogen that reproduces profusely when we eat sugar and grains. Candida infections are epidemic today, and we do not know how to treat it with any degree of success.

As a fetus in your mother's womb, you're microbe-free. Then, as you make your way down the birth canal, you begin to acquire the millions of bacteria that make up your biome. This is one reason mother's milk is so important to babies: newborns pick up good microbes from the breast milk as well as from the skin around the nipple, which become part of their intestinal flora. Later, more microbes enter your gut as you begin to explore the world—sucking your toes, being kissed by your parents and licked by the family dog, stuffing food into your mouth with filthy fingers. A microbiologist friend recently suggested that the reasons humans kiss is so our bugs can test to see if they're going to get along!

And while we have a dozen or so square feet of skin, we have more than 3,000 square feet of gut surface—that's approximately the size of a tennis court. Our gut is constantly tasting the environment through the foods we ingest. In fact, the primary way we engage with the world is through our gut, not our hands or skin or digital devices. The GI tract won't work properly unless we have enough variety of the right flora. But every time we take an antibiotic we are "nuking" all the gut flora, the friendly as well as the bad, decimating their population, but not touching the Candida, that then happily proliferate.

Later in this book you are going to learn how to repair your gut and eliminate Candida using probiotics that you prepare at home.

The Toxic Effects of Candida

In nearly every kitchen cupboard you will find a most deadly toxin: sugar. The typical American adult consumes 150 pounds of added sugar a year, including high-fructose corn syrup and fake sugars like aspartame, saccharine, and sucralose.[3] Processed grains are major sources of the sugar we consume. Even foods we don't think of as sweet—like catsup, peanut butter, and yogurt—often contain sugar or sugar substitutes. That delicious Greek yogurt you had this morning and you think is so healthy may contain more sugar than a can of soda pop. So be sure to always check nutrition facts and ingredients lists for hidden sources of sugar!

You may think that putting Splenda in your tea is a healthier choice than using natural sugar, but artificial sweeteners can be even more harmful. Fake sugars confuse your brain by making you crave something to eat even when you're not really hungry. And then you satisfy your cravings with sugars and grains, the very foods that feed Candida in the gut and lead to weight gain.

Sugar in all forms (except honey) also reduces your levels of brain-derived neurotrophic factor (BDNF), a hormone that triggers the growth of stem cells in the brain and repairs crucial brain structures. Some experts believe that the connection between diabetes and Alzheimer's—a hot topic these days—is attributable to the typical Western diet high in sugar.[4]

Food cravings aren't just a psychological problem, all in your head; they're in your gut. You may think that you're gorging on chocolate cake or tortilla chips because you love the taste, but the real reason you can't eat just one is that the Candida in your gut thrive on sugar, and to get their fix they release chemicals that bring on carb or sugar cravings. When lab rats that have become addicted to cocaine are given a choice between cocaine-laced water and a sugary soda pop, they invariably choose the soda pop.[5] Sweets excite the same centers in the brain that are stimulated by drugs like heroin and cocaine. They release the neurotransmitter dopamine, triggering a pleasure response, so you associate the food with pleasure. Then, wanting more pleasure, you eat more of the food. The cycle continues, and you become addicted to comfort foods. And the food companies know this!

There are no known benefits to the human body of Candida. The job of Candida is to ferment your body after you die so it decays properly. What an elegant solution nature came up with for disposing of the carcasses of the dead! As your body decays, proteins and fats begin to break down and become food for Candida. You do not want this to happen a day too early.

Athelete's foot can be caused by Candida overgrowth, and women are familiar with vaginal infections caused by this yeast. Most doctors continue to treat it as a localized problem. In reality, when Candida makes its way into the vagina or infects the toenails it is an indication that it is also abundant in the gut in its pathogenic fungal form. (Candida has a harmless "commensal" state and a harmful fungal state. Indeed, the same microbes that can cause life-threatening diseases are often harmless inhabitants on our mucosa until they begin to grow out of control and upset the balance of the colony.) Whenever you give in to your cravings and reach for a cookie or a breakfast muffin or a plate of pasta, remember the *Candida albicans* are winning the battle for your gut.

Candida, with its 6,000 or so genes, is huge in comparison to the good bacteria in your gut, with their 28 or so genes. Antibiotics will decimate the bacteria in your gut but do not affect the yeasts. After a course of antibiotics, the Candida proliferate, often creating biofilms they can hide under. They move into the best real estate in your gut—they occupy all the good apartment units and take over all the parking spots. And later, when you swallow a little probiotic, hoping it'll replenish your gut flora, and it comes along asking the Candida to move out, the Candida is going to laugh at it. Imagine walking into a biker bar and asking one of the leather-clad Hell's Angels to move off his barstool so you can have a seat!

To reclaim your gut for the good bacteria, you have to eliminate the bad guys, the Candida. Otherwise all of the probiotics you consume will end up going straight into the toilet, because there is no place for them to move into. Doctors will sometimes prescribe an antifungal medication, as this class of medicine will kill the yeasts but not the good bacteria. This creates another problem, however. The dying Candida begin to secrete toxins that result in brain fog, flu-like symptoms, and even fever and body aches. Then, you have to deal with the corpses of trillions of dead yeast inside you. This is called a Herxheimer reaction, or die-off reaction.

Counteracting Candida with *S. boulardii*

The secret Candida buster is a friendly yeast called *Saccharomyces boulardii*, or *S. boulardii*. This is a noncolonizing, nonpathogenic yeast strain that competes with Candida and displaces it, moving the Candida through your GI tract and out in your stool without killing it. *S. boulardii* is sensational because it remains inside you only for five or six days before being eliminated naturally. There is no die-off effect. Within two weeks you will have cleared a major portion of the Candida in your GI tract. During this time, you must be taking a quality multi-strain probiotic so that the good bacteria can move in and colonize the newly available real estate in your gut. (I offer specific recommendations for superprobiotics in Chapter 6.)

You might be unfamiliar with *S. boulardii*, but it has a track record as a probiotic spanning more than 60 years. A company called Florastor sold more than 11 billion doses in the United States. The yeast was discovered in 1923 by anthropologist Henri Boulard, who isolated the strain from the skin of lychees and mangosteen in Southeast Asia. You can buy it separately from any other probiotics.

You are already familiar with the Saccharomyces family, as the *cerevisiae* strain, commonly known as brewer's yeast, is used to ferment beer and bake bread. The difference is that the *S. boulardii* strain simply passes through your GI tract in less than a week, competing and driving out the bad Candida in the process. In taking *S. boulardii*, you will also be getting the benefit of the metabolites, the powerful by-products it manufactures. (Another example of metabolites from yeast is beer, from *S. cerevisiae*.) I believe that the metabolites are actually as powerful as the *S. boulardii* yeast itself, and provide great benefits. According to research, *S. boulardii* also dramatically reduces the population of the bacteria *H. pylori* in the gut to levels where they do not cause peptic ulcers or cancer.[6]

As remarkable as *S. boulardii* is, you can't just take a few capsules and expect miracles. In fact, the reason you do not find many manufacturers adding *S. boulardii* to their probiotics is that it causes gas and bloating if you have a lot of sugar in your diet. The *S. boulardii* aren't going to fight Candida if there is a slice of birthday cake in your gut. Instead, they're going to have a feast eating the chocolate-chip cookies and fries that you just had for dinner. Then you will feel bloated and uncomfortable and find yourself passing gas. You should not take *S. boulardii* when you have lots of sugar in your system.

A powerful strategy for eliminating Candida is ingesting *S. boulardii* after two or three days of avoiding sugars and processed grains. *S. boulardii* is nontoxic, and unless you have HIV or are immune compromised, it does not remain inside your body. Also, it poses little danger of fungemia, a phenomenon where the yeast ends up going into the bloodstream. *S. boulardii* is even used with premature babies, as it has been shown to prevent the growth of pathogens, including *Escherichia coli,* or *E. coli.*[7]

The power of *S. boulardii* depends on the dosage. And here is the crux of the problem: Most *S. boulardii* you buy in a health-food store has been grown in a lab and fed white sugar and then transported over great distance under changing temperature conditions. In other words, it's not happy. The microorganisms that survive are hibernating inside a gelatin capsule, and the last thing in the world that they want to do is to wake up in a stomach full of acid. These warriors arrive in your gut half-asleep and starved. They are no match for the Candida terrorists that have been feasting and growing strong inside you.

The solution is to grow your own *S. boulardii* at home using our recipe (see page 241). The *S. boulardii* you cultivate will be much more potent than the store-bought variety, and will be growing on high-quality sugars from your favorite organic fruits. Your *S. boulardii* will be ready in two or three days, after it transforms all the sugars into potent metabolites. When the fermentation process ends, the *S. boulardii* will go dormant. At this point you want to place your brew in the refrigerator and take a full soupspoon every morning before breakfast for two weeks.

Now you will be ingesting a very alive formulation with billions of *S. boulardii* yeasts ready to go to work displacing the Candida in your system. I like to think of *S. boulardii* as the U.N. Peacekeepers that go into troubled parts of the world to clear out the bad guys. You want to prepare them to do their very important job, so start growing this Candida-busting yeast while continuing to avoid all sugars and grains. You should take this in the morning when you do not have any sugars in your gut, in order to avoid bloating.

In our Center for Energy Medicine in the Chilean Andes, we have batches of *S. boulardii* that go back many generations, each new batch becoming stronger and more intelligent than the previous one as a result of our prayers and intention. I have seen cases of parasites cleared up in a one-week course of *S. boulardii.* When I travel to Asia or to the Amazon rain forest, I always carry

S. boulardii capsules with me, because while they are not as powerful as the ones I grow at home, they will stop traveler's diarrhea in children or adults in a matter of hours. If you can prepare this probiotic at home, you'll begin eliminating the stubborn Candida and prepare your gut to host a broad range of beneficial microbes. This is an essential step for you to grow a new body.

Dealing with Environmental Toxins

Environmental poisons make up an overwhelming percentage of the toxins in our bodies. We have been assaulted by pesticides, industrial chemicals, preservatives—even antibiotics and birth-control medication flushed down the toilet that makes its way into the community water table. A U.S. Geological Survey study showed that estrogen in rivers and waterways are resulting in increasing numbers of fish with "intersex" characteristics—males with immature female egg cells in their testes.[8] There are over 80,000 industrial chemicals in use today that were unknown 100 years ago. Burning fossil fuels and disposing of manufacturing waste have added even more contaminants to our living environment, which find their way to our dinner plates and drinking water, increasing our toxic load.

Our ancestors were largely protected from such challenges. For thousands of years, the earth was able to accommodate changes brought about by human intervention. Our impact on the land we roamed over and the waters we fished was minor, creating no permanent damage to the ecosystem. We lived sustainably: our food was organic, our waste was easily recycled, and we built homes of natural materials like mud and straw. We didn't have genetically modified foods, or plastic bottles with a half-life of 10,000 years, or nail polish laced with formaldehyde.

All that changed, however, as we started to mine products like lead and mercury, and introduce them into our homes—and bodies—through everyday products like paint, bathtubs, light bulbs, lead pipes, and dental fillings, and more recently through contaminated fish and seafood. Mercury is a known neurotoxin, and both lead and mercury have been implicated in developmental problems like learning disabilities and ADHD. (The expression "mad as a hatter" is said to refer to the mental disorders suffered by millinery workers who were exposed to mercury vapors in the manufacture of felt hats, a common practice in the 18th and 19th centuries.) Metals like lead and mercury are stored in body fat, including the fat that makes up 60 percent of the brain.[9]

Heavy metals are not the only toxins that impact our health. In the last century or so, we've released thousands upon thousands of man-made chemicals into the environment. Molecules synthesized in the laboratory are in everything from pesticides, clothing, shampoos, nonstick cookware, electrical appliances, and plastic water bottles to chemicals used in mining and manufacturing, and even in drugs. Data on how these chemicals affect us are scarce: of the 82,000 chemicals approved for use in the United States, only a quarter have been tested for their effect on humans. But none of these molecules can be safely ingested by insects or bacteria and then recycled into a substance that the human body or the environment can use. (There's a reason fast-food French fries don't lose their color or shape when they sit for months underneath a car seat in the family SUV: no self-respecting microbe would have anything to do with such toxic food.)

The regrettable consequence is that most of the chemicals we manufacture remain in the environment. Even pristine lakes in the Swiss Alps are contaminated with sludge that includes mercury, cadmium, and lead, the residues of waste from decades past before these toxic elements were banned or restricted. We have older buildings filled with lead-based paint, and carcinogenic chemicals are contaminating the bottom of rivers that flow past polluting factories. Pharmaceuticals we toss in the garbage or flush down the toilet join the mix of toxins in the earth, water, soil, and air. Among the most ubiquitous contaminants in the U.S. are flame retardants, which saturate virtually everything manufactured. Flame retardants are surface coatings: as microscopic particles flake off, they bind to dust and are circulated through the air. Researchers have found flame retardants in an array of popular foods on the supermarket shelves, including butter and peanuts. Even more disturbing, they've found flame retardants in mother's milk.

And we humans are not the only beings affected. Killer whales that recently washed up in the Georgia Strait were so filled with PCBs (polychlorinated biphenyl, a group of chemicals banned in the U.S. in 1979) and other toxins that the whales were declared a health hazard and treated as toxic waste.

The human brain is not designed to handle the toxins released into the environment over the last century. This is not news for many of you reading this book. What *is* new is our understanding that these neurotoxins prevent us from attaining the experience of Oneness so easily reached by our Paleolithic ancestors.

I tell my students that we are all born with a bucket inside each of our cells, where we deposit toxins we have collected during our lifetime. Some of us are born with a bigger bucket while others have a smaller one. Once your bucket is full and starts to overflow, you end up with symptoms of disease. This is when Western medicine intervenes, treating pathology. But what we want to do is to empty the bucket regularly, before disease appears. When our bucket is full of toxins, our cells are not able to repair and regenerate. We are unable to grow a new body.

Genetically Modified Foods

The havoc we've created with man-made chemicals may be matched by another even more insidious threat found in the foods we eat every day. Some of the toxic overload in our guts comes from genetically modified foods. In most cases, we don't even realize toxins are on the menu. Scientists are increasingly altering the DNA of crops to create products that will last longer, be more resistant to disease and pests, and look and taste better.

Plants can't flee from their enemies, so nature equipped them to synthesize chemicals that act as natural insecticides to repel predators. But more than 90 percent of the corn grown in the

U.S. contains a genetically modified gene that allows the plants to produce an even more powerful insecticide. Bugs that attempt to eat the corn are killed instantly as their stomachs burst open. The gene spliced onto corn—and cotton crops—is from *Bacillus thuringiensis* (Bt) bacteria. The food industry claims that Bt toxin poses little threat to humans or animals—it is rapidly destroyed in the stomach, they say. Yet mice exposed to Bt have shown dramatic effects, from allergic reactions to intestinal damage.[10]

Bt toxin is now found in nearly 85 percent of all streams and waterways in America, and more than 90 percent of pregnant women tested showed Bt toxin in their blood.[11] Clearly Bt isn't cooperating with the industry's claims, increasing the likelihood that it will be around long enough to have lasting effects on our food supply.

Soybeans are another crop that are almost entirely genetically modified. Monsanto's Roundup Ready Soybeans are engineered to tolerate the pesticide containing glyphosate. Scientists are now finding that the genetically modified proteins in corn and soy may be inserting their genes into the DNA of the friendly bugs in your intestines, where they continue to function long after you've stopped eating the soy or corn.

Genetically modified tomatoes, squash, and sugar beets are commonplace today. And we find genetically modified foods not only in the produce aisle but also in sections of the supermarket where we would least suspect, like the fish department—from fish that have been farm raised on genetically modified corn. In fact, more than 70 percent of all foods on the grocery store shelves contain a food substance that has been genetically altered. Unless you eat foods clearly marked "Certified organic by the USDA," you are taking part in a genetic experiment that is unprecedented in Earth's long history.

Toxic Effects of Grain

Genetic engineering isn't the only danger from food that can harm the gut-brain. Globally, we're faced with new diseases caused by our grain-based diet. The problem is that the wheat we're eating is not the wheat people ate even 75 years ago. To eliminate famine in the Soviet Union, the post–World War II green revolution introduced a high-yield drought-resistant dwarf wheat containing 20 times more gluten than the old European strains, changing the composition of the bread we're eating. (Gluten is a protein that gives dough its elasticity.) The dramatic increase in celiac disease—an autoimmune disorder in which ingesting gluten damages the gut lining—and gluten sensitivity is related to this major change in our diets.

Zonulin is a protein found in wheat that was discovered by gastroenterologist Alessio Fasano and his team in the year 2000.[12] Zonulin will pry open the tight junctions between cells in the lining of the gut, allowing food particles and gut bacteria to enter the blood and triggering a local immune response, as bacteria do not belong in our bloodstream. It seems that the human body does not recognize zonulin, and that gluten-sensitive individuals have elevated levels of zonulin in their bloodstream, even though they have not been diagnosed with celiac disease. And Fasano believes that *no* human being completely digests gluten.

The human digestive system hasn't evolved to function well on a grain-based diet. Whether or not you're among those who suffer from celiac disease, the harsh truth is that we *all* have become gluten intolerant to a surprising degree. This may be due to the fact that grains are a relatively new addition to the human diet, and the decimation of our intestinal flora by antibiotics may be compounding our difficulty in digesting gluten. Grains have become toxic to many of us, and our grain-rich diets continue damaging the gut.

When the brain is fueled by sugars from grain, it reverts to a primitive, predatory survival mode, adversely affecting our emotions and overall health.

Toxins from Within

Not all of the toxins affecting the gut-brain come from the environment. Toxins are also produced by parasites in the gut and by the breakdown of hormones. These toxins are called endogenous because they originate inside you. The microbes eat and eliminate waste just as we do, and endogenous toxins they produce can affect the brain.

Henry Lin, a researcher at the University of Southern California's Keck School of Medicine, has mapped out a new way of thinking about how toxins in the gut affect the brain. According to Lin, wayward bacteria migrating from the large intestine into the normally bacteria-free small intestine can create a bacterial imbalance.[13] This triggers a response in the immune and nervous systems that can lead to insomnia, anxiety, depression, and impaired cognitive function. Serotonin levels drop. What Lin describes is common: small intestinal bacterial overgrowth (SIBO) affects thousands of people in the United States. It can be resolved with a combination of *S. boulardii* and a diet free of sugars and starches.

What Happens in the Gut Doesn't Stay in the Gut

It's clear that what happens in the gut affects the whole body. A healthy gut is filled with trillions of friendly bacteria that help you digest food, synthesize vitamins B and C, and help reduce cellular inflammation that can lead to disease. They also play an important role in creating and maintaining the mucosal immune system in your gut. They even train your immune system to identify pathogens—the microorganisms that make you sick.

The good bacteria are supposed to far outnumber the bad bacteria in the gut, but too often, grains and sugar disturb the balance of your flora. Hormones, antibiotics, and other drugs in nonorganic meat, poultry, and dairy also encourage the growth of yeast and bad microbes. An increasing number of people are diagnosed with a debilitating form of colitis known as *Clostridium difficile*, or *C-diff*, that's linked to antibiotic use. People on antibiotics are 7 to 10 times more likely to get *C-diff* while on the drugs and during the months afterward.

People diagnosed with *C-diff* can be helped by ingesting fecal matter from healthy individuals. It sounds disgusting, but if you were in danger of losing your life due to a severe and debilitating intestinal infection, my guess is you would get over any squeamishness. A study published in the *New England Journal of Medicine* in January 2013 reported a 94 percent cure rate of *C-diff* when administering fecal transplants, compared to just 31 percent with the potent antibiotic vancomycin.[14] Someday there may be options to help some of the half a million Americans a year who get *C-diff.*

Most of us aren't ill enough to need such a radical overhaul of the microorganisms in our GI tract, but nearly everyone shows signs of an imbalanced gut—although we may not link gas, bloating, joint pain, mood swings, mild depression, and allergies to problems with our digestive flora.

If we avoid gluten and processed wheat, breads, and pasta, and rebuild our flora with good-quality probiotics, the digestive system will gradually restore the colonies of friendly microorganisms and eliminate or limit most of the unfriendly ones. But if we continue eating gluten-laden foods, the result is most likely to be inflammation, decreased immunity, and a condition known as leaky gut syndrome.

Your flora are not only in your gut, they are in your mouth, nose, and skin. It's important to protect the health of your entire biome, not just your gut. Showering with chlorinated water will kill the good flora on your skin, so get a good water filter for your house or at least your bathrooms. And be cautious, as using mouthwash will eliminate the good bacteria in your mouth that prevent gum disease.

Perils of a Leaky Gut

The lining of the intestines is only one cell thick, and the gluten in grain can loosen the tight junctions in the gut wall. If the wall becomes permeable, or "leaky," undigested food fragments and bacteria can slip through the gut lining and into the bloodstream. Imagine a net made of stretchy material that becomes more permeable as it stretches. As more foreign matter reaches the bloodstream, the condition worsens.

Your body treats the gluten protein like an invading parasite. This sets off an autoimmune reaction, releasing chemokines and cytokines, the chemical messengers of the immune system, which instruct killer T cells to attack the gut lining. The result is food sensitivities, rashes, joint pain, and inflammation throughout the body. Meanwhile, the liver and kidneys go into overdrive to process the toxins in the bloodstream. With so many poisons circulating in the blood, many of these end up passing through the blood-brain barrier, a protective membrane designed to prevent toxins in the bloodstream from getting into the brain.

The effect of leaky gut syndrome on the brain can be dramatic and far-reaching: headaches, brain fog, poor concentration, and short-term memory loss are common symptoms. (Many so-called senior moments are due to leaky gut.) Some people will experience depression or anxiety. Others become hyperactive, impulsive, and short-tempered. The toxic load on the brain disables the higher circuits for love, beauty, creativity, and joy.

Through all this, you struggle to understand why you're so moody, or why you keep misplacing your cell phone, or why your world seems more hostile and threatening. In this condition, you have absolutely no chance of experiencing the higher states of consciousness.

The best way to repair a leaky gut and reverse the toxin overload that leads to it is twofold: eliminate sugar and gluten from your diet and replenish the friendly intestinal bacteria. Like I said earlier, replenishing the friendly flora in your gut is a two-step process. First you prepare the terrain with S.

boulardii, flushing out the Candida and parasites. Second you take a high-quality probiotic. This should contain a variety of strains and be potent—at least 50 billion CFUs (colony forming units). (For specific recommendations, see Chapter 6.)

Detoxifying from sugar requires cutting out not just the obvious sugary foods but also processed grains, which turn into glucose instantly, spiking your blood sugar and feeding your Candida. Whole grains contain enough fiber to keep blood sugar levels steady, but if you want to upgrade your brain, you'll need to avoid *all* processed grains during your seven-day Grow a New Body program, before reintroducing small amounts of whole grains. If this seems unnecessarily strict, note that the minimum daily requirement of *processed* carbohydrates is zero.

Eliminating sugar also involves cutting out fruits like watermelon and raisins, which have a higher glycemic index than a candy bar. Fruits and vegetables that are high in fiber slow the absorption of glucose, so your blood sugar doesn't spike. I encourage you to become familiar with the glycemic index of your favorite foods so you can make the best choices for yourself.

Next you will learn how to switch on the longevity genes hidden in your DNA code.

Chapter 5

SWITCHING ON THE LONGEVITY GENES

We spent many millions of years feasting and then fasting. When food was abundant, nature turned on reproduction. Females became fertile, and both males and females buffed up and put on muscle mass and stored fat reserves. When times were lean, nature sensed our survival was threatened by possible starvation—females became infertile and all the repair and regeneration systems were turned on, ensuring our survival until more abundant times.

If we can create the conditions that mimic starvation, while keeping ample nutrients on board, we can trigger the DNA switches that allow us to grow a new body.

Intermittent Fasting

Abstaining from food for short periods as a way to cleanse body and mind has a history going back millennia. Indigenous medicine men and women, Buddhist monks, Christian mystics, and others would subsist on only water for a few days to prime the brain to function optimally and pray. In the process they would repair and upgrade their body. However, there's no need to fast from good carbs, including fruit, for more than 18 hours at a time. Brain repair starts to happen quickly, and brain fog begins to clear in a matter of days. Even during Ramadan, the month-long period of fasting that is one of the most sacred practices of Islam, Muslims fast only from sunrise to sunset each day. As long as you drink plenty of water and refrain from rigorous exercise while you're fasting, you may find that you don't even experience hunger pangs, or if you do, that they're mild enough not to bother you.

One form of intermittent fasting involves not eating any grains, or anything that turns into sugar in your bloodstream between 6 P.M. and noon the next day. This daily 18-hour fast will bring you into ketosis, a metabolic change that happens when your cells exhaust the energy from carbohydrates and sugars, and break down fats into a powerful fuel known as ketones. Then your brain starts burning ketones for fuel.

Ideally, you will follow this fasting routine for the rest of your life, or at least for as long as you wish to keep your vibrant health. Before you do the three-day vision quest in Chapter 14, where you will drink only water, you should reduce the toxins in your system by practicing the daily 18-hour fast and being able to cycle in and out of ketosis easily for at least three months.

Hunger pangs while fasting are good; they are an indication that you're switching from the glucose fuel to the ketones, and your brain is beginning to burn fats. But your ancient limbic brain, that runs on sugars, may try to convince you that you'll die if you don't eat a glazed doughnut right away. Don't give in to it. Simply observe your cravings, knowing that in fact, your body has enough fuel reserves to get you through the next 40 days without eating—though I don't recommend it!

"Hanger" pangs are different. Hanger is what happens when you become angry as you get hungry. If you find yourself getting hangry as you do the daily 18-hour fast from sugars, it is because of Candida overgrowth in your GI tract. They want to be fed, and want to be sure that you know this, and they begin releasing toxins that signal the brain to increase the levels of ghrelin, the "hunger hormone."

The purpose of intermittent fasting is not for weight loss. That's a dangerous misuse of the practice. You fast in order to go into ketosis and turn on the body's fat-burning system and repair mechanisms. Fasting brings about detoxification at a cellular level. Reducing the intake of sugars and processed carbs for more than a few hours triggers a process called autophagy, in which more than 90 percent of the "waste" inside the cells is recycled into amino acid building blocks the cells can reuse for repair, and the remainder is eliminated as garbage. Cells have a most efficient recycling system. If our cities were as effective in recycling waste as our cells are, we would hardly have any garbage in our landfills.

As you detox, you release cellular waste into your bloodstream, where it's carried to the GI tract and to the liver to be flushed out of the body. But fasting can be dangerous if your liver is not working properly, because if you are not eliminating the toxins in your bloodstream, you are *recycling* them. And the worst place toxins can end up in is the fatty tissue in the brain.

When Eastern sages and Western Christian mystics fasted, they did not have to deal with a toxic burden in their body or brain that modern humans have. They were not exposed to the chemicals you find today in our foods, in cosmetics, in water, and in the air. The Chernobyl nuclear tragedy had not contaminated the air and gardens in Europe, and the Fukushima Daiichi nuclear disaster had not contaminated the waters of the Pacific Ocean and the seafood that ends up on our dinner plate.

Upon entering ketosis during fasting, their bodies would go into repair mode, and they would activate higher order neural networks in the neocortex. They would begin to grow a new body as they attained mystical Oneness.

When we're burning carbs, the body is in building mode; insulin levels are high as we build muscle. When we stop utilizing carbs as our primary fuel, even for a few hours, we go into ketosis. This allows the body to recycle waste and repair itself. It triggers the production of stem cells in the brain and every organ in the body. It also awakens the higher order neural networks where we can have a spiritual experience, even when we are not looking for one.

Even during a short fast, amazing things happen to the body and brain. In just 24 hours, the production of human growth hormone increases by 1,500 percent, repairing cells that make up our tissues. Not eating carbs for as little as 18 hours switches on the longevity genes.

Intermittent fasting should be done carefully if you are hypoglycemic or diabetic. You should not undertake any long-term fasting until your blood sugar levels are regulated. Do not attempt this program while trying to maintain a diet made up primarily of sugar-filled, processed carbs. This means that you need to eliminate the pizza, pasta, bagels, croissants, potato chips, soda pop, and so on before starting this program. Be sure to fill your diet with high-fiber vegetables, avocado, olive oil, coconut oil, and raw nuts.

The payoffs of the 18-hour daily fast are as follows:

- **Increasing your metabolism.** After you exhaust the sugars in your bloodstream, your cells will begin to burn fat for energy.

- **Providing a quality fuel for your higher brain.** The ketones (fats) are jet fuel for the brain and will switch on the higher order neural networks involved in creativity, discovery, exploration, compassion, and the experience of Oneness necessary to grow a new body.

- **Lowering levels of insulin.** When you lower the levels of glucose in your bloodstream, your need for insulin is reduced, because insulin's job is to remove glucose from the bloodstream. Insulin receptors in the cell have a chance to reset and reduce insulin resistance, and the risk for diabetes.

- **Increasing the detoxification of every cell in your body.** Ketosis allows for autophagy and recycling of cellular debris, emptying out the garbage.

- **Preventing cancer and reducing the proliferation of existing cancer cells.** While cancer cells can readily burn glucose (sugar) for fuel, their impaired metabolism makes it difficult for them to burn ketones (fat). In addition, ketosis lowers the levels of the tumor marker IGF-1. That is a sign that the ketosis is preventing cancerous tumors from growing or spreading.

- **Protecting the brain.** Ketosis reduces inflammation in the brain and body and turns on the production of stem cells in the brain. It does this by activating BDNF, brain-derived neurotrophic factor, which enhances brain repair.

Be sure that you give your liver support for eliminating the toxins that will be released into your bloodstream from your fatty tissues as you begin to burn fat for fuel. Zinc, B12, magnesium, and glutathione will help your liver do its job. Without these nutrients, the liver will not eliminate toxic waste effectively, and the toxins may end up in your brain.

Two Meals a Day

Who said that we need to eat three meals a day, that breakfast, lunch, and dinner are necessary or desirable? Our nomadic hunter-gatherer ancestors ate whenever they got hungry (and had food available), and so did the Native Americans when Europeans first arrived in the New World. Abigail Carroll, author of the book *Three Squares: The Invention of the American Meal*, explains that the Europeans believed their regular eating habits and "civilized" mealtimes distinguished them from the "grazing" practice of the natives, a habit they associated with animals.

How wrong they were about timing your eating!

Ditch the three-meals-a-day-plus-snacks habit that we have been accustomed to. If you are interested in growing a new body, you need to think of a new golden rule of eating only one or two meals a day, and skipping breakfast (and sometimes dinner). I prefer skipping breakfast rather than skipping dinner because it draws out the period of recycling and ketosis provided by intermittent fasting. You can eat organic, plant-based, nutrient-dense, and calorie-poor foods until full during the six-hour window.

It will take a few weeks to persuade your gut flora to become comfortable with eating only one or two meals a day. Remember that they are the ones who eat first, and you have trained them to eat three meals a day or more. Once your body has shifted into fat-burning mode, you will find it easy to go for 18 hours without feeling hunger pangs. Your cravings for sugars will gradually dissipate as you eliminate the Candida and you restart your fat-burning engines that have been dormant for decades.

Some bugs in your gut will not like this at all, particularly Candida that you have rewarded with sugary treats for years. So prepare your homemade *S. boulardii* and have it ready to take every morning!

How Much Protein Do We Really Need?

Humans and animals have co-existed side by side for a long time. We have been domesticating sheep, pigs, and cows before the dawn of agriculture, and have been eating animal products, including dairy and meat, since then. Even in our hunting and gathering days, our ancestors would feast on a lucky find of eggs. Granted, our Paleolithic forebears had meat infrequently, as they had to hunt it or fish for it; however, for the last few thousand years, animal protein has been a staple of the human diet.

Today meat is at the center of one of the world's bloodiest food fights. Most of the meat consumed in the developed world comes from factory farms where animals are treated with extraordinary cruelty, fed hormones and antibiotics, and raised in unsanitary and inhumane conditions. But healthy, organic, grass-fed meat in small portions and wild-caught fish can foster freedom from heart disease, diabetes, cancers, and dementia.

Although we need protein, our cells actually cannot use protein. Our gut bacteria must break it down into amino acids, which are the building blocks of proteins. If your gut flora is damaged, you will not get the necessary amino acids. Amino acids cannot be stored, and the ones that are not used promptly get converted into glucose or fat, then burned for fuel.

There are many amino acids found in nature, but humans can only use 20 of them for building proteins. *Essential* amino acids are the ones you need to get from food, because your body cannot make them. *Nonessential* amino acids are the ones your body makes on its own.

Protein makes up about 33 percent of the weight of a piece of beef, so if you eat a 100-gram steak you are only getting about 33 grams of protein. Lentils, meanwhile, have 9 grams of protein per 100 grams. In contrast, salmon has nearly 25 grams of protein per 100 grams. A good general rule for most people is to limit your total protein intake (animal and plant-based) to 200 to 400 grams or less per week, depending on your weight. Your body does not need protein every day. Eat your protein, especially animal protein, on a cycling schedule, largely abstaining from protein on the days in between.

Remember to feast and then fast!

If you are looking at these recommendations and thinking, *You've got to be kidding. My body wants more meat than that!*, it's likely your gut flora is damaged and you are not absorbing amino acids properly. The more damaged your gut is as a result of antibiotic use or age, the more protein you may require.

The key to animal protein is high *quality*, not high quantity. When we eat meat, we need to be concerned about what the animal ate too. Meats from animals that are not raised on the foods nature intended for them are not the best protein source. After all, animals did not graze on the corn that they are fed in the factory farms of today. Make sure that your meat is free range, grass fed, and vegetarian. Wild-caught fish are better than farmed fish, which are fed cereal.

Most important, forget about your daily protein intake, and think about weekly protein intake. Remember that our ancestors were hunter-gatherers who ate all their protein at once when they had a good day of hunting. They feasted and fasted, cycling their protein consumption.

The key is cycling protein. I consume about 300 grams of protein a week, which is perfect for my weight (165 lbs, or 75 kg) and level of activity (moderate exercise). And I will eat most of my protein on days one and four of the week, in two sittings, just like our Paleolithic ancestors did when they found a fresh mammoth on their way home and shooed the birds away and brought it back to the village—except that instead of mammoth, I will eat a couple of hard-boiled eggs at lunch and a portion of fish in the evening.

So Sunday and Wednesday, I will have a protein feast, maybe eating out at my favorite fish restaurant or having a double scoop of plant-based protein powder at lunch or a helping of black beans and rice, which is a typical Cuban dish and a complete protein.

I am on the road teaching and lecturing a lot, and I often have to go to dinner with the hosts of my program. If the night before I had a big protein meal, I know that my mTOR is activated, so that evening I will have a soup and salad with no animal protein, to again silence mTOR. (I explain mTOR in the next section.)

The key is cycling protein.

I know that what I'm telling you flies in the face of our current popular beliefs about our protein needs, but stay with me. Years ago, I was a fervent advocate of restricting carbs. Now that new research has come out and I have experienced for myself the benefits of restricting protein intake, I am convinced that eating less protein is key to growing a new body and to sustaining health and longevity. I believe that many Paleo dieters are exposing themselves to increased risk of cancer and degenerative disease because of excessive protein intake.[1]

Protein and Evolution

To understand our basic food requirements, we have to go back to when life first appeared on Earth.

Around 2 billion years ago, the first bacteria appeared on Earth. Their mission was to eat and reproduce. When there was lots of food available, they grew strong and multiplied. When food was scarce during times of starvation, nature turned off reproduction and all their resources went into repair and survival. These early bacteria needed a way to determine if there were abundant nutrients for reproduction or if they needed instead to conserve energy, using scarce food supplies to repair in preparation for a time when food would be more plentiful. This protein-sensing system is known as TOR (target of rapamycin), and it is shared today by all creatures from bacteria to whales to humans. You'll learn more about TOR and its very important work shortly, but for now, know this: Consuming too much animal protein stimulates the TOR pathway, which can cause out-of-control growth of cancer cells. Cancer cells want to multiply quickly.

Why would our bodies be controlled by a process that could end up killing us? Remember that nature selects for the longevity of the *species*, but not of the individual. It wants us to reproduce so that our species doesn't become extinct—and if you happen to die on the way to the species surviving, nature shrugs. Your challenge is to work with your natural intelligence to continue to enjoy good health and live long past your reproductive years. Restrict your protein intake and quiet TOR, and your chances of living a long and healthy life improve immensely.

For a species to survive, birth rates need to be higher than death rates—and this has to happen even when there are times of extreme hardship. But nature will not allow any animal to reproduce if there is danger of famine or starvation. That's because carrying and nursing offspring, as mammals do, requires a lot of energy and takes a huge toll on the mother, who must feed herself as well as the young she is carrying. When we practice intermittent fasting (with adequate nutrition) our body focuses on repair and renewal. We literally trick the brain into thinking that there is danger of starvation and that its resources should go into growing a stronger and more resilient body.

The Grow a New Body program works by calibrating the level of TOR in your system!

During times of food scarcity, many creatures will go into a dormant state so they can wait out the long winter. We see this in bears that hibernate and in yeasts found in the skin of grapes. As winter approaches, a yeast cell will "sleep." When food supplies become available again in the spring, TOR will sense an abundance of nutrients, and it will "wake up" again. Some bacteria can even withstand boiling and freezing temperatures, and endure many years of extreme weather, before the TOR system detects the right nutrient conditions for germination. And while most of the genes of the yeast on the skin of the grape go dormant, the TOR nutrient sensors remain alert, ready to rouse the organism when there are adequate nutrients in the environment.

As I mentioned, humans have a TOR system, just as yeast do, and it's called mTOR ("m" is for mammalian).

On the Grow a New Body program, you won't be fasting for months, just hours, to get a similar result.

Now that we understand the science behind mTOR, we know we can make dietary choices that downregulate it (restricting protein) and effectively send our bodies into repair and longevity mode.

How TOR Works

In periods of famine, women will become infertile—mTOR makes sure their bodies do this, and male sperm counts will go down dramatically. During this time the resources in the body are dedicated to eliminating toxins through autophagy, switching on the longevity genes, and silencing the genes that create disease, all of which are fantastic strategies for long-term survival, until food sources become plentiful again. Humpback whales fast for many months in the tropics, losing up to half of their body weight and clearing diseases evident on their skin. When their bodies have repaired, they migrate north where food is abundant and switch into reproduction and growth mode.

The TOR sensors detect the presence of amino acids and sugars. Billions of years ago, when the first bacteria were feeding on the amino acids found in the young earth, some developed the ability to use light as a food source. These were the first cyanobacteria, or blue-green algae, and they discovered photosynthesis—how to feed on sunlight. These early plants turned light and minerals into carbohydrates, and thus the first sugars appeared on the earth in significant quantities. These plants would become the food of the large herbivores that later walked the earth.

The earliest sources of energy (food) in the earth were amino acids, which are the building blocks of proteins and sugar. The TOR sensors measure the abundance or scarcity of these two foods. When things were good, TOR stepped on the reproductive accelerator. When food was in short supply, it put on the brakes on having babies or cells dividing and switched on the long-term survival systems. For humans it meant recycling cellular waste to capture 90 percent of the amino acids from damaged proteins, and maintain steady amino acid levels in the blood.

To summarize, we can think of our all-important TOR as the "brain" that senses nutrients and that controls growth and longevity in all animals. When we avoid sugars and reduce proteins, TOR instructs our cells to go into repair and longevity mode. Stem-cell and antioxidant systems that protect the brain and all cells are activated. And you prevent or delay the appearance of cancer and the proliferation of existing tumors.

THE DISCOVERY OF mTOR

Rapamycin, a drug used to prevent rejection of transplanted organs, comes from a bacterium discovered in 1960 on Easter Island. Doctors were surprised to find that patients taking Rapamycin had a reduced incidence of cancer despite the fact that the medication they were taking suppressed the immune system, which the body depends on to kill cancer cells. It turns out that rapamycin was downregulating mTOR (the target of rapamycin).[2] This causes the body to go into repair and longevity mode, and inhibits rampant cellular replication, which is the hallmark of cancer. We are learning that downregulating mTOR through intermitent fasting is a key to preventing cancer and helping the body repair.

Debunking Other Dietary Myths

The only proven strategy for extending both life span and health span in mice and primates by up to 30 percent is reducing the total number of calories they consume, primarily the carbs that turn into glucose.

We know a low-carb diet will keep insulin levels in the body low. Combining that with a high-protein intake was thought to be the key to extending the life span of all the animals on a calorie-restricted diet. But it turns out that the longer life span was due to a protein called IGF-1, or insulin-like growth factor-1, a growth factor we need when we are young and are growing fingers and toes. But for adults, high levels of IGF-1 are associated with pathological growth—it indicates the likelihood of a cancerous tumor present or developing. As you lower your IGF-1 levels, you reduce your chances of developing cancer.

When blood sugar levels are high, IGF-1 tells mTOR that there is lots of food available, and mTOR shuts down repair and switches on cell growth. Therefore, the key to longevity is lowering sugar *and* protein intake.

The New Science on Diet

It turns out that long-term caloric restriction does not actually lower IGF-1, but *protein* restriction does.[3] You can eat organic steaks, keep your blood sugar levels low, and be in mild ketosis, burning fats instead of sugars for energy—and this combination will allow you to feel great, lose weight, clear the brain fog, and have tremendous energy. But mTOR will still be activated from eating too much animal protein. Overeat meat and you will not be flipping the genetic switches to grow a new body; instead, you will be opting for an early death even as you tone and strengthen your muscles.

Amino acids are detected by mTOR directly. They do not need IGF-1 or mediating hormones to do the job. In a recent research study, Roberto Zoncu and his colleagues at the Massachusetts

Institute of Technology stated that "a significant advance in our understanding of the regulation and functions of mTOR has revealed its critical involvement in the onset and progression of diabetes, cancer and aging." Clearly, it's important to not just avoid sugars but to also avoid overeating protein. The authors conclude that "recent findings suggest that mTOR signaling controls the rate at which cells and tissues age, and that inhibiting mTOR may represent a promising avenue to increase longevity."[4]

A high-protein, low-carb diet is great for weight loss and for achieving a toned beach body, which is one of the key reasons this type of diet became popular. Unfortunately, it is not very good for long-term health. The bottom line is that eating too much protein accelerates aging and the onset of cancer. Meat and eggs should be a side dish rather than the main course. I personally eat about 8 ounces of fish during the week, and a couple of eggs once or twice weekly. I generally avoid red meat, but will have a bison steak once in a while or a small fillet of grass-fed free-range beef.

The Crux of the Matter

The solution turns out to be far simpler than we thought. The proteins that activate mTOR seem to be the branched chain amino acids (BCAAs). There are three BCAAs: leucine, isoleucine, and valine. And they are found predominantly in animal products, including red meat, dairy, cheese, and eggs.

Luigi Fontana and his colleagues at Washington University in St. Louis, Missouri, demonstrated that "a moderate reduction in total dietary protein or selected amino acids can rapidly improve metabolic health in both humans and mice. Reduction of dietary protein or total amino acids decreases fasting blood glucose levels and improves glucose tolerance in both species in less than six weeks."[5]

The verdict is in. The culprit is animal protein.

So what's the bottom line: how much animal protein should we eat?

Very little is the best answer I can come up with. It seems that the staples of the Western diet, meat and dairy, are partially to blame for the tremendous increase in obesity, diabetes, heart disease, and cancer.

Valter Longo, Ph.D., a cellular biologist at the University of Southern California, found that starving a mouse receiving chemotherapy or other targeted therapies will protect normal cells and organs while making the therapy up to 40 percent more toxic to cancer cells. In human clinical trials, Longo found that periods of no food for two to four days at a time during a six-month period killed older and damaged immune cells and triggered the generation of new healthy ones. "We could not predict that prolonged fasting would have such a remarkable effect in promoting stem cell–based regeneration," explains Longo.[6]

Fasting forces the body to use stores of glucose and fat as well as breaking down white blood cells. This depletion of white blood cells triggers stem cell–based regeneration of new immune system cells. Fasting reduces the enzyme PKA that extends longevity and is linked to the production of stem cells and pluripotency—the potential for one cell to become many different cell types. Fasting also lowered levels of IGF-1, the growth factor associated with tumor progression and cancer risk.

Longo explains: "PKA is the key gene that needs to shut down in order for these stem cells to switch into regenerative mode . . . and the good news is that the body got rid of the parts of the system that might be damaged or old, the inefficient parts, during the fasting. Now, if you start with a system heavily damaged by chemotherapy or aging, fasting cycles can generate, literally, a new immune system."[7]

Protein restriction is the key. And be sure to avoid the protein bars that are full of sugar and the packaged protein powders. Make vegetable proteins and legumes your main source of good amino acids.

It's important to note that legumes contain lectins; these are anti-nutrients, proteins that can bind to sugars. These compounds reduce the body's ability to absorb minerals from your food. So when you prepare legumes, soak them overnight and rinse them well. I like to ferment them overnight with *S. boulardii*, to further neutralize the anti-nutrients they contain. (Instructions for overnight fermentation are in Chapter 6.)

The Truth about Carbs

When it comes to "cheap carbs," the worst offenders are the simple carbs in processed foods that turn to sugar right away in your gut. A slice of white bread, for example, raises your blood sugar more than a spoonful of white sugar. If you are running your system on sugars, you are using a short-lived energy strategy. The body stores glucose as glycogen, and you can only store about 100 grams of glycogen in your liver. This is enough for a 20-minute work-out at the gym! Your muscles can store about 400 grams, enough for 90 minutes of endurance exercise. But the average 165-pound man in good physical shape has close to 55 pounds (25 kg) of stored fat he can use for energy, which is nearly 1,000 times more fuel than that glycogen in his liver!

The complex carbohydrates in broccoli, cauliflower, and asparagus are long molecules of glucose that your gut bacteria break down into sugars. However, complex carbs do not spike your insulin, so they do little damage; they are also nutrient rich, packed with phytonutrients necessary for good health. In addition, vegetables appear to quiet the mTOR sensors.

Choose your vegetables and fruits for color. Be sure to include two or three dishes of vegetables every day. And it is best to eat your fruit during lunch so you can burn the sugars during the afternoon and go into ketosis, burning fats into the night and the morning.

You may be wondering, *If I have to go lean on carbs (even healthy ones) and low on protein, what the hell do I eat?*

For starters, *fat.*

The Skinny on Fat

Most of your calories should come from fat. When you eat a high-fat and low cheap-carb diet without excessive proteins, you enter into nutritional ketosis, so your body will be burning fats for fuel rather than glucose. If you are like most people, it will take a few days for your body to remember how to burn fats, as you have been running your metabolic engine on sugars for a long time. But once you switch on the fat-burning furnaces, you will notice that the brain fog will begin to clear, your muscle mass will increase, and you will naturally start losing weight. As your insulin levels drop and you lower your intake of proteins, you will be downregulating mTOR and reducing inflammation, and your levels of leptin (the anti-hunger hormone) will stabilize, reducing your food cravings.

When you switch over to burning fats, you turn on your cell's recycling systems, or autophagy. I like to point out to my students that probably the most important workers in New York City are the garbage collectors. If you go for a walk through Manhattan late in the evening, you will see stacks of garbage bags piled on the sidewalks. Yet by morning they are all gone, and the streets are clean again. Imagine what would happen if the garbage collectors went on strike even for a few days! Autophagy is the garbage collection (and recycling) in the body. And for many of us that have been living on a sugar-rich diet, the garbage collectors inside us have been on strike for many years. Consequently, cellular waste has accumulated inside and outside our cells, and broken-down proteins have not been recycled.

By reducing carbs and consuming the right amount of proteins, you turn down the volume on mTOR and switch on autophagy. Voilà! The strike is over, the workers return to clean up the garbage, broken proteins are recycled—which reduces the need for dietary intake of proteins—and you begin to grow a new body.

Figure 5.1 shows how it works.[8] Let me walk you through it.

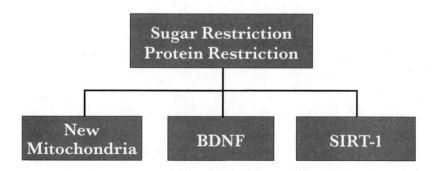

Figure 5.1: The benefits of protein and sugar restriction

When you limit your intake of carbs and proteins, you have three incredible, measurable benefits. The first is that you trigger the production of new mitochondria, the fuel factories in every cell in your body. That phenomenon is known as mitochondrial biogenesis.

The second benefit is that you increase your levels of brain-derived neurotrophic factor (BDNF), which switches on the production of stem cells inside the brain. A few decades ago we did not believe that the brain could regenerate or that we could grow new neurons. Today, we understand that we can activate the growth of new neural stem cells that repair and upgrade the brain by turning on the production of BDNF. It also reduces your levels of a death-promoting protein, BAX, associated with neurons dying in your brain. This may be important in preventing Alzheimer's and other forms of dementia.

Last, and perhaps most important, reducing carbs and proteins will switch on the SIRT-1 genes: these longevity proteins silence the genes that create disease and wake up the genes that create health. I like to think of the SIRT-1 family of genes as the immortality genes. And they are only active when you eat a low-carb, low-amino acid diet. In a high-carb, high-protein environment, the SIRT-1 genes go silent.

The key to receiving all the benefits I have just described is not only eating more fats—such as avocados and the coconut oil, olive oil, and grass-fed butter that you use to prepare and enhance your meals—but burning your own fat through ketosis.

Even if you are not particularly interested in losing weight, you want your body to run mostly on fats rather than sugar. As you are cranking up your metabolic engine, you can help the process by adding good fats to your diet, including coconut oil, olive oil, avocados, and so on. But you do not want all of your fats to come from these outside sources, or you will not be turning on autophagy. The garbage inside cells will not be cleared away, and the recycling of amino acids will not be as effective as when you are burning your own fat stores.

Your body in its great wisdom will not allow you to burn your own fat stores until you eliminate the toxins that are stored there. Remember that the body stores toxins in fat tissue. In your fat, you may have the residual mercury from your own and from your mother's dental fillings and from the time you played with mercury at the age of eleven when a thermometer broke; pesticides in the food you ate as a child; lead from the lead pipes in your home or coming in from the street; and aluminum from cooking pots (or the aluminum foil you cooked with). All of these are stored in your fat tissue, together with the endotoxins, or internally created toxins, including the products of incomplete breakdown and elimination of spent hormones. Your fat tissue has been holding on to all of that for a long time.

If you are thinking that burning fat sounds good but eating fat doesn't, you should know that government guidelines have been revised in 2015 to no longer limit the amount of fats or cholesterol in our diet. Saturated fats, found commonly in coconut oil, dairy, and meat products, were once maligned and blamed for heart disease being the number one killer in America. Today we know that there is no link between them and heart disease.

In fact, the higher the amount of saturated fats that you consume, the better for your brain and your health. These are anti-inflammatory, are stable, and do not oxidize easily. (Oxidation is the process involved in steel rusting, copper turning green, and a cut-open apple turning brown.)

Fats do not cause a spike in blood sugar or trigger the release of IGF-1. That means they don't upregulate mTOR. Instead, they contribute to quieting it.

The Truth about Fat

Here's the skinny on the different types of fats:

Saturated fats: The best are the MCTs, or the medium-chain triglycerides, which are used quickly by the body and do not go into storage in fat cells. The best MCTs are found in coconut and olive oils, as well as butter and avocados. MCTs are jet fuel for the brain, and supplementing with them during the Grow a New Body program will help keep your mind clear as your body starts to burn its own fat reserves. It will provide a great transition until you begin to produce ketones from your own fat stores.

You might be wondering: Aren't coconut oil and other saturated fats bad for you because they raise cholesterol? Turns out that the fats that cause heart attacks are the ones that come from eating sugar and carbs, not from eating fat. Remember that your liver converts excess sugars into fat. In effect, the role of insulin is to convert sugar into fat—the sugar our ancestors ate at the end of summer when the fruit was ripe for all of six weeks was stored as fat to help take them through the long winter. The saturated fats protect against heart attacks, and come from animal products like cheese and butter. Saturated fats are essential for our immune system. They raise LDL cholesterol, but they also increase HDL ("good" cholesterol) while sugar lowers HDL. While coconut oil is 40 percent saturated fat, people from countries that consume the most coconut oil seem to have the lowest rates of heart disease on the planet.

As you are relearning to burn fats for fuel, you may want to help your system with a mixture of MCT oil (made from coconuts) and coconut oil. A tablespoon of each in the morning is a great way to kick-start your fat burning. The MCT oil provides ketones immediately, while the coconut oil turns into ketones gradually, fueling you throughout the day. Repeat two to three times daily as needed.

Monounsaturated fats (MUFAs): MUFAs are your good friends. They are found in olive oil, avocados, nuts and nut oils, olives, and butter.

Polyunsaturated fats (PUFAs): PUFAs can be good and bad. The two most important ones are omega-3 and omega-6. Omega-3 reduces inflammation, switches on the production of stem cells in the brain, helping to repair the memory and learning centers, and protects you from heart disease. Omega-6 is pro-inflammatory, so you have to be careful with this fat.

Before we lived in cities, our prehistoric ancestors consumed omega-3 and omega-6 in a ratio of 1:1. Today our processed foods provide us with nearly 20 times more omega-6 than omega-3. In the Lyon Diet Heart Study, more than 300 subjects and an equal number of controls were followed for four years. Researchers found that decreasing the amount of omega-6 the people consumed and increasing the omega-3 fat intake resulted in 70 percent fewer heart attacks, reduced the overall mortality rate, and protected against cancer.[9]

Omega-3 fatty acids are abundant in avocados, grass-fed meat, flaxseed and flaxseed oil, and fatty fish like salmon. And you should supplement with 2 to 3 grams of omega-3 daily.

Trans fats: These fats are the problem! A few decades ago, hydrogenated oils (trans fats) replaced butter in processed foods in a misguided effort to lower the consumption of saturated fats. We now know that these fats contribute to dementia, inflammation, and diabetes and increase the risk for cancer. Avoid anything that says "hydrogenated" in the label!

Stay away from any of the seed and vegetable oils, including corn oil, soybean oil, canola oil, sunflower oil, and margarine. Instead, choose organic, cold-pressed, extra-virgin olive oil. You can pour it directly on your food, including salads, fish, and cheeses like fresh mozzarella. You cannot eat too much of it, but do not cook with it, as it has a low smoke point. (Cooking with oils above the temperature of its smoke point causes the creation of toxins and free radicals.) Use coconut oil in your smoothies, to make a vegetable stir-fry, or to cook with, as it has a high smoke point.

Serve fats with every meal! And remember, although fats go great with veggies, a sure way to put on weight is to add in starches and sugars—plus, you will raise your bad cholesterol.

Chapter 6

SUPERFOODS AND SUPER SUPPLEMENTS

Be very, very careful what you put into that head,
because you will never, ever get it out.

— Cardinal Thomas Wolsey, about King Henry VIII

Enjoying the superfoods and the Grow a New Body supplements in this chapter can all but eliminate your risk for Alzheimer's, cancer, diabetes, and a host of other diseases of civilization.

Wild versions of many superfoods formed the basis of our earliest ancestors' diet and continue to be central to the diet of many indigenous people today. In the few hunter-gatherer societies that still exist, autism, dementia, diabetes, cancer, and autoimmune disorders are very rare or nonexistent. Not coincidentally, the diet in these societies has changed little in centuries. Nuts, berries, fruits, vegetables, and small game served as our ancestors' primary food sources long before grain became a dietary staple. Today, most of us live farther away from nature than hunter-gatherers do, and we purchase our food at farmers' markets or grocery stores rather than forage in the wild. But we, too, can come close to the ideal diet that supports growing a new body if we understand what it includes and why it's so beneficial.

Anthropologists long ago abandoned the idea that meat from hunting big animals was central to the early hunter-gatherer diet. Humans co-evolved with the plants, not the animals, and for thousands of years, we were incredibly awkward hunters. (Imagine trying to bring down a large beast with a rock or a stick.) Even after early hunters developed spears 500,000 years ago, animals in the wild could easily outrun them and often outsmart them. Buffalo or mammoth meat was only a rare adjunct to a mostly plant-based diet that included protein sources like nuts, seeds, and insects, and on occasion, fish and small game. When a great creature was captured, it was considered an offering from Spirit.

Some 50,000 years ago, we became more skilled at the hunt. But by then we had been consuming nuts and berries and greens for a couple of million years, and the animals were considered sacred, their lives were not to be taken lightly. Take the origin of the word *animal*. It comes from the Latin *anima*, meaning soul. Humans also belong to the animal world, and wild creatures were our sacred relations. Before Columbus came to the New World, there were more than 60 million bison grazing in the Great Plains of North America, but by 1890 there were fewer than 200 left in the United States. Reckless hunters had caused a near extinction: a popular sport of the time was shooting these great creatures from the back of a passenger train while crossing the plains and leaving the carcass to rot on the ground. Indigenous people, by contrast, never hunted for sport, and when they killed an animal, they used every bit of it: the meat for food, the hide for clothing, the sinew for building materials, and more.

Starting around 6,000 years ago, agricultural-era humans changed their primary food from wild greens to grains they cultivated in their fields. Depending on where they lived, wheat, corn, or rice became their dietary staple. All of these grains are a major cause of high blood sugar. Essentially, they started fueling their bodies and brains on glucose.

By now every schoolchild knows the value of green plants in the diet. What most of us don't realize, however, is that plants provide vital intelligence to the body beyond simply ensuring a balanced diet. Scientists have found that plants are master regulators of our genes. MicroRNAs, or MiRNAs—single strands of plant genetic material—circulate through our bloodstream, switching genes on and off.[1] These microscopic vegetable strands regulate our cholesterol levels and direct the destruction of invading viruses and bacteria. MiRNAs are the ultimate social networkers, sending messages quickly to individual genes. Like the Nrf2-rich plants (but using other pathways), they have the power to switch on the genes that create health and to switch off the genes that create cancer, heart disease, diabetes, and many of the other ailments of civilization.

In over 30 years of clinical research at the University of California Medical Center, Dr. Dean Ornish has found that a primarily plant-based diet will activate more than 500 disease-preventing genes and deactivate more than 200 disease-causing genes. While Dr. Ornish's program includes whole grains as part of the plant-based diet, I recommend cutting out grains altogether during the seven-day Grow a New Body program. This will lower your blood sugar to the point of switching on autophagy and downregulating mTOR. After that, you can add in some whole grains slowly, observing whether your body tolerates them well.

The Grow a New Body program relies on juicing leafy green vegetables in the morning. For millennia a plant-based diet was standard fare for humans, yet most of us aren't used to having green juices, salads, and vegetable soups for breakfast. The Green Goddess Juice you will drink to break your fast each day will direct the repair of every organ in your body and restore brain health. The codes activated by the greens will switch on repair systems in the entire body.

Most green vegetables have a very low sugar content, so even when you juice them, removing most of the fiber, they won't spike your blood glucose. You can have your fiber-rich veggies later. Fiber does slow absorption of sugar and helps digestion, and feeds friendly bacteria in the gut. Be aware that root vegetables like beets and carrots are high in sugars and low in fiber, so they're not recommended during the Grow a New Body program, although you can add them back into your diet later in moderation.

Some plants are considered superfoods because of the epigenetic instructions they provide to your DNA. Phytonutrients are the reason the villagers I met along the Amazon did not suffer from the four great maladies of modern life: cancer, heart disease, diabetes, and dementia.

Cruciferous vegetables, tomatoes, and various nuts and seeds are central to the diets of people who live in blue zones—areas around the globe where the inhabitants have unusual longevity and good health, most notably Okinawa, Japan; Sardinia, Italy; Nicoya, Costa Rica; Ikaria, Greece; and Loma Linda, California, which is home to a large community of Seventh-day Adventists, a religious group that maintains a lacto-ovo vegetarian diet (a vegetarian diet that includes dairy products and eggs).

As a rule of thumb, the more colorful a fruit or vegetable, the richer it is in phytonutrients and the greater its power as a superfood. While we can also ingest phytonutrients in the form of nutritional supplements, eating them in their natural form lets us get the full benefits of their living nutrients.

No matter how carefully we think we're eating, we may still be missing out on nutrients, however. Research indicates that much of the produce found in supermarkets is relatively deficient in phytonutrients compared to produce sold at farm stands and farmers' markets or picked from your kitchen garden. And even farm-fresh produce can't match the power of its wilder cousins. As Jo Robinson, author of *Eating on the Wild Side: The Missing Link to Optimum Health,* explains, "Wild dandelions, once a springtime treat for Native Americans, have seven times more phytonutrients than spinach, which we consider a 'superfood.' A purple potato native to Peru has 28 times more cancer-fighting anthocyanins than common russet potatoes. One species of apple has a staggering 100 times more phytonutrients than the Golden Delicious displayed in our supermarkets."[2]

The reason for this nutrient loss, Robinson explains, is that for the last 10,000 years, farmers have been selecting the sweetest, least bitter plants to grow in their fields and orchards, selectively breeding out the sour taste of most wild foods. Today we understand that the bitter, astringent flavor of some vegetables indicates that the plant is high in polyphenols that protect the plant—and you—from disease. But our farming ancestors selected plants that were high in sugar and low in fiber—quick energy sources that were tastier. The result was a steady decline in the health benefits of plants we used as food.

For maximum benefit, we should eat vegetables and fruits that are in season, free of pesticides, and locally grown. The fruits and vegetables that most grocery stores sell as fresh are picked days or weeks before they're ripe, with the idea that they'll ripen in transit. In the process, they lose much of the flavor and nutritional value they would have gained from ripening naturally under the sun. Think of how flavorful a garden-fresh tomato is, and how bland and papery its grocery-store cousins taste. Supporting local farmers not only ensures that our produce will be fresh but also reduces the carbon footprint of transporting foods long distances.

If good, fresh fruits and vegetables aren't available locally, the best alternative is frozen organic produce: frozen fruits and vegetables are picked at the height of freshness and immediately flash-frozen. Canned fruits and vegetables should be avoided at all costs. These processed foods contain all sorts of chemicals and other unhealthy additives, and much of the nutritional value has been lost. Whenever the opportunity to gather wild foods presents itself, go for it. Nothing tastes quite like a salad of wild dandelion greens!

The Nrf2 Activators

Among the holy grail of the superfoods are the cruciferous vegetables, which include broccoli, cauliflower, cabbage, and kale. (*Cruciferous* doesn't refer to a property of the vegetables but rather to the petals of the plants, which grow in the shape of a cross.) High in fiber and antioxidants as well as phytonutrients, cruciferous vegetables activate the Nrf2 protein inside cells and turn on the SIRT-1 longevity genes.

Nrf2 is able to protect every organ in the body and every kind of tissue against diseases like cancer, heart disease, dementia, and autoimmune disease. It is one of the most important cellular defense systems, designed to eliminate free radicals and oxidative stress produced by toxins and carcinogens. (A free radical is a molecule that has lost an electron, making it unstable. It will try to steal an electron from another molecule.)

When Dr. David Perlmutter and I were examining certain plants used by Amazon peoples, we found that many of them are Nrf2 activators. The Nrf2 protein is normally bound to the cell membrane until it is activated by stress, caloric restriction, or by certain plants, including garlic, broccoli, turmeric, and other superfoods. Newly freed from the membrane, it enters the nucleus of the cell and sets to work, switching on the production of antioxidants, detoxifiers, and anti-inflammatory agents. Figure 6.1 gives you an idea of how Nrf2 works, and some of the foods and substances that will trigger it to action.

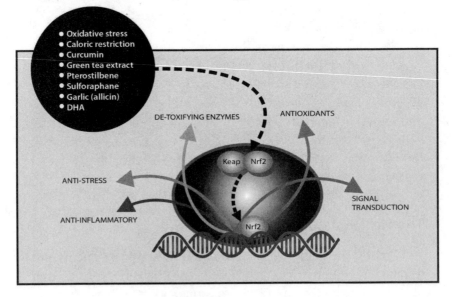

Figure 6.1: The Nrf2 detox pathways

I like to think of Nrf2 as the U.S. Navy SEALs, who are normally in a military base drinking coffee (or green tea) until they are called to action and then go into the nucleus of the cell and into the DNA, cleaning up the terrorists (free radicals) and switching on the SIRT-1 longevity genes. When their job is done, they return to the cell membrane and remain on alert.

Researchers have found that Nrf2 might be the master regulator of the aging process. Scientists at the University of Texas claim that "the Nrf2-signaling . . . activates more than 200 genes that are crucial in the metabolism of drugs and toxins, protection against oxidative stress and inflammation, as well as playing an integral role in stability of proteins and in the removal of damaged proteins via proteasomal degradation or autophagy."[3]

How did the shamans of old know about this master regulator of longevity found in select green plants? Obviously, they asked the plants themselves.

Luckily, today we can find the best Nrf2 activators right in our local health-food store. But we must know how to use these powerful plant medicines. You can eat as much broccoli as you like every meal, but you cannot take the Nrf2 activator sulforaphane, which comes from broccoli florets, for more than a week without overloading the very systems you want to switch on. Similarly, you can prepare curry every day with turmeric and experience its great health benefits: People in India where a lot of curry is consumed only have 15 percent of the Alzheimer's risk that Americans have. But you can take curcumin, the active ingredient in turmeric, for only one week, and then let the body rest.

To keep it simple, you can eat the whole plant as much as you like. However, the plant extract, the active ingredient, has a *dose-dependent* effect. This means that a little bit will help you, but a large amount will shut down the beneficial effects. This effect is known as *hormesis* (from the Greek "turning on"). This is the case with all Nrf2 activators—a low dose can help you, and a high dose can reverse all their benefits. After a few days of turning on the Nrf2 response with broccoli extract (sulforaphane), or curcumin from turmeric, the body will saturate and turn detoxification off, making you sick with your own waste!

The following are the most powerful plant activators of Nrf2 and regulators of the aging process.

Cruciferous Vegetables	
Bok choy	Cauliflower
Broccoli	Collard greens
Brussels sprouts	Kale
Cabbage	Mustard greens

Broccoli originated in the Mediterranean and is mentioned in ancient Roman texts. Commonly used in Italian cooking, it first came to America when Thomas Jefferson brought it from Europe. Broccoli is usually green, but there's a purple variety as well. You can eat both the stems and florets. Broccoli can be steamed, baked, roasted, grilled, or chopped up and eaten raw in a salad. It can also be used in a soup or casserole, although you'll want to avoid thick, creamy soups and cheesy casseroles, which contain dairy. Broccoli is rich in calcium, selenium, and zinc, among other nutrients. Broccoli is high in sulforaphane, a powerful Nrf2 activator. Sulforaphane has anticancer properties and ups the expression of the longevity genes inside cells.

Cauliflower originated in both Europe and Asia. It is usually white, but there are also purple and orange varieties. Packed with nutrients and high in fiber, cauliflower is often used in Indian curries and roasted with the spice turmeric, another phytonutrient. Like broccoli, cauliflower can be steamed, baked, grilled, or eaten raw, and can be used in a soup or casserole.

Cabbage and **Brussels sprouts**, recognizable by their heads of tightly packed leaves, are loaded with nutrients. In fact, cabbage was used in ancient Greece and Rome to remedy myriad illnesses. Brussels sprouts are rich in folic acid and vitamins A and C, but if undercooked they have a bitter taste that makes them the least favorite vegetables in the cruciferous family. Grilled or baked, they are very tasty.

Bok choy, or white cabbage, is a staple of Asian cooking. Cultivated in China for over 6,000 years, it is now grown in North America as well. Nutrient dense, bok choy contains a whopping 28 phytochemicals,[4] including one found to prevent ovarian cancer.[5] It's high in vitamins A, C, and K and folate. Bok choy is also a good source of calcium, as unlike spinach it is low in oxalate, a substance that binds to calcium and makes it unavailable to the body. Bok choy can be eaten cooked or raw, and is a healthy addition to a green juice.

Kale, like spinach and other greens that don't form a head, has become wildly popular in the West—deservedly so. It's packed with fiber and phytonutrients, and is a good source of vitamins C, K, and beta-carotene, as well as calcium and magnesium. I have kale every morning in my green juice. The bluer the color, the more nutritious it is.

Collard greens have a phytonutrient content that's off the charts. They may be the most effective of the cruciferous vegetables at reducing the risk of cancer and cardiovascular disease. Among the oldest members of the cabbage family, collard greens were popular in ancient Greece. They came to America from Africa with the slave trade and are such an integral part of traditional Southern cooking that South Carolina declared collard greens the state vegetable. They can be cooked in a variety of ways, and their wide leaves can be used like bread or tortillas as a wrap for guacamole.

Mustard greens, which can be red as well as green, have a peppery taste resembling arugula's. Phytonutrient superstars, mustard greens are second only to Brussels sprouts in cancer prevention. For maximum nutritional benefit, chop the greens, and then let them sit for five minutes before cooking.

Turmeric

Along with all the healthy veggies that are central to the Grow a New Body program's eating plan is **turmeric**, a spice loaded with health benefits. A key ingredient in curry, turmeric is important for detoxification and brain repair. It is an extremely powerful anti-inflammatory, antioxidant, antifungal, and antimicrobial. Turmeric's health benefits are optimized when it's cooked, but it can also be combined with black pepper and taken as a food supplement.

Derived from the root of the *Curcuma longa* plant, turmeric is said to enhance sexual desire and was traditionally used in marriage rituals in India and Tamil.

Turmeric has an earthy, strong flavor and, when dried, a deep yellow-orange color that suggests a connection to the life-giving power of the sun.

Nuts and Seeds

Nuts and seeds are excellent sources of healthy, plant-based fats. Oils from coconuts, walnuts, almonds, and flaxseeds are, like extra-virgin olive oil, concentrated sources of omega-3 fatty acids and confer a long list of health benefits, from lowering cholesterol to lifting depression.

Among **nuts**, walnuts are phytonutrient superstars, but other varieties also have significant talents. Almonds are high in fiber. Brazil nuts contain selenium, a cancer fighter. Two Brazil nuts will give you all the selenium you need for the day. Cashews are rich in iron, zinc, and magnesium, a brain booster. Pecans help prevent plaque from forming on the arteries. Macadamia nuts contain the most monounsaturated (good) fat of any nut. Peanuts—technically legumes, not nuts—are packed with nutrients, but it's best to avoid them. Many people are sensitive to peanuts, and full-blown peanut allergies are common—and can be fatal.

Seeds are another good way to up your protein and omega-3 essential fatty acid intake. Hemp seeds, with ten essential amino acids, are an excellent protein source, and they contain omega-3 and omega-6 fatty acids in an ideal ratio. Sesame seeds are high in calcium and other minerals. Sunflower seeds promote healthy digestion. Pumpkin seeds contain cholesterol-lowering lignans and aid digestion by regulating the passage of food from the stomach to the small intestine.

Both nuts and seeds can be sprinkled on salads, included in vegetable dishes, or eaten plain. To get the most nutritional value out of nuts and seeds, be sure to buy unroasted, organic ones and store them in the refrigerator to keep them fresh and prevent mold.

Avocados

The ancient peoples of the Americas knew that the fruit of the avocado tree was a superfood offering a host of benefits. Don't be put off by the high fat content: avocados contain healthy monounsaturated fats including oleic acid, which lowers the risk of breast cancer and increases nutrient absorption in the gut. Avocados are a good source of lutein, a carotenoid that prevents macular degeneration, and of folic acid, a B vitamin that prevents heart disease and strokes. High in fiber with a low glycemic index, avocados help regulate blood sugar. They're also a good source of the antioxidant glutathione, and when paired with spinach or tomatoes, which are high in alpha-lipoic acid, pack a one-two punch that protects cell health. Guacamole, made with avocados, tomatoes, parsley, and a little lime, salt, and onion, makes a phytonutrient-rich dip. Just don't grab a bag of tortilla chips for dipping: use cut-up raw vegetables instead.

Berries

Blueberries are phytonutrient rock stars, containing pterostilbene, an Nrf2 activator that lowers cholesterol and blood pressure and protects against cancer and dementia. Among the few fruits native to North America, blueberries were a dietary staple of Native Americans across the northeastern U.S. Known for their antioxidant properties, blueberries are also rich in iron, selenium, and zinc. If you can find the wild variety, grab them: their nutrient value is even higher. I favor the frozen ones that are picked at the height of ripeness.

Goji berries, also known as wolfberries, are native to China, where they've been touted for centuries as the key to long life and are a staple of Chinese medicine. Nutrient dense, the berries contain two to four times the antioxidant properties of blueberries, as well as all essential amino acids, making them a whole protein source, like meat. Generally, you would eat goji berries raw or brewed in a tea or cooked in soup, for medicinal purposes, but you can also use goji berry extract.

What to Eat in Moderation

Ancient humans didn't have access to fruit year-round, so their bodies adjusted to eating only the fruits that grew where they lived, harvested in season. Except in tropical climates, *in season* meant when the fruit ripened at the end of the growing season—usually the end of summer. From an evolutionary standpoint, the role of insulin—the hormone produced by the pancreas to signal cells to absorb sugar—was to turn these fruit sugars into fat that was stored by the body, to provide energy for our hunter-gatherer ancestors throughout the long winter. Today, however, the long winter with few food sources never arrives, so we're stuck with excess fat, typically in the midsection.

Since we haven't evolved to eat fruit after the growing season, consuming too much of it throws off the insulin system and hyper-activates mTOR. Therefore, eat only a moderate amount of fruit, consuming it as whole fruit, not juice, to prevent blood sugar spikes and get the full benefit of the fiber. If fruit is out of season, but you *really* crave it, try eating a few frozen blueberries or sprinkle a small amount of dried berries, grapes, or cherries onto a salad.

The exception to the no-juice rule is the green drink to start off the day. Avoid premixed green drinks sold commercially;

most are just sugary fruit juice with a little kale or spinach added to color them green. Making your own juice with fresh leafy green vegetables will give you a lasting infusion of vitamins and micronutrients, including those that turn off the genes for disease and turn on the genes for health.

As you begin the seven-day Grow a New Body program, keep in mind that avocados, nuts, seeds, and eggs (unless you're allergic to them) are good sources of protein. Avoid red meat while on the program, but after that, as you start to upgrade your gut-brain, you can eat animal protein in moderation. In a study of 6,000 Americans, Dr. Valter Longo showed that consuming a high-protein diet is associated with a 75 percent increase in overall mortality and a three- to four-fold increased risk of cancer, in contrast to a low-protein plant-based diet.[6]

There is a lot of misinformation about getting all your proteins from greens. The American Heart Association states that plant proteins are deficient because most lack one or more essential amino acids. And if you lived your entire life eating only broccoli, you would be missing out on some essential amino acids. But the moment you prepare two or three servings of different vegetables, you are getting all the essential amino acids your body requires. The only thing that vegetarians would be missing and need to supplement is vitamin B12.

If you are going to eat meat, however, find the cleanest free-range meat and poultry you can; animals allowed to graze with other animals and consume a natural, plant-based diet are high in omega-3 fatty acids.

When our ancestors left the African savannah for the coast, they incorporated fish and mollusks into their diet. All over the world, civilizations sprang up around oceans, lakes, and rivers. Emperors, governors, and high priests dined on shellfish, mollusks, and fish, while their pyramid-building subjects were fed wheat and bread. Today fish is within the reach of most everyone who lives near seafood-rich waters or can open a tin of sardines.

Packed with the omega-3 essential fatty acid DHA, fish is a superior brain food. Avoid farmed fish, which are often pumped full of antibiotics and supplements to enhance color, and fed soybeans and grain that they would never eat in the wild. The wild varieties—especially cold-water fish like Alaskan wild salmon, sardines, and herring—are lower in toxins. But bear in mind that the larger the fish, the more likely it is to be contaminated with mercury, so avoid tuna and swordfish.

The DHA-rich fish oil was so highly prized by North American Indians from the Pacific Northwest, that it was traded like currency. The "fat" in the so-called candlefish was so rich in oil that you could simply stick a wick in the mouth of one of the dried fish, and it would burn like a candle![7]

Fermented Foods

Fermentation is an ancient method of food preparation going back to at least 8000 B.C.E., and you can find fermented foods in every part of the world. Based on culturing friendly bacteria, fermentation produces everything from wine, beer, and cider to bread, cheese, and vinegar. Fermented foods provide essential enzymes and probiotics that repair the gut and help rid the body of toxins, including heavy metals.

My favorite fermented foods are pickles, sauerkraut, and miso soup. You can find excellent recipes for fermented foods on the Internet, as well as how-to videos on the culturing process. If you're going to ferment foods yourself, just make sure to follow the directions carefully, to avoid contamination from unwanted bacteria.

Fermentation is a way of preserving food and maximizing its health benefits, using naturally occurring bacteria to convert sugars into lactic acid. Sally Fallon and Mary G. Enig, Ph.D., of the Weston A. Price Foundation, which disseminates research and information on nutrient-dense foods, explain how fermentation works:

> *Starches and sugars in vegetables and fruits are converted into lactic acid by the many species of lactic-acid-producing bacteria. These lactobacilli are ubiquitous, present on the surface of*

all living things and especially numerous on leaves and roots of plants growing in or near the ground. Man needs only to learn the techniques for controlling and encouraging their proliferation to put them to his own use, just as he has learned to put certain yeasts to use in converting the sugars in grape juice to alcohol in wine.[8]

OVERNIGHT RICE FERMENTATION WITH *S. BOULARDII*

During our Grow a New Body programs, we ferment many foods, including rice, with *S. boulardii*. If you place two capsules of this amazing yeast in brown rice and soak overnight, the *S. boulardii* will neutralize the anti-nutrients in the rice and turn it into a superfood with powerful anticancer properties that reduce the growth of lymphomas.[9]

To prepare, simply use two cups of water for one cup of rice. The water should be at body temperature. Open two capsules of *S. boulardii* (or one tablespoon of starter from an earlier homemade batch) and place the contents in the water and stir. Leave overnight in the oven with only the oven light on, to maintain body temperature. Remove about 1/2 cup of water the following day and cook in the remaining water.

You have now prepared your own superfood! You can use the water you removed as your starter for the next batch of rice that you prepare.

Prebiotics and Probiotics

Prebiotics and probiotics are essential for upgrading your gut-brain.

Prebiotics promote the growth of good flora in your gut. Cruciferous vegetables have been called prebiotics because they contain fiber that your flora feed on, serving as the latticework and the food for good bacteria. To upgrade your brain and keep it functioning optimally, you need to consume plenty of plant fiber, or roughage. Fiber speeds the movement of food through the digestive system by absorbing water, which softens stools, making bowel movements easier.

Probiotics are the healthy flora that facilitate digestion and protect the gut against harmful microbes. We ingest many bacteria in our ordinary interactions with the natural environment, whether it's by inhaling dust that rises from the soil as we garden, or by petting a dog or cat, or simply by holding another person's hand. In fact, there are myriad ways we bring healthy organisms into the body, ranging from handling organic fruits and vegetables before rinsing off the soil to swimming in a lake or stream. A single gram of earth—about the size of a small coin—contains over 40 billion bacteria. To upgrade your gut-brain, spend more time outdoors, or get a dog!

If you don't feel you're getting enough probiotics in the ordinary course of your life, you can take a supplement. The best I've found are the "smart" probiotics that my friend Compton Rom Bada, a microbiologist, has gathered from the five longevity regions around the planet. (You can order his ProAlive Probiotic at ascendedhealth.com.) Compton's intelligent probiotics can repopulate the flora in your gut in a matter of weeks, whereas off-the-shelf formulas that contain dead or inactive flora aren't as effective. Remember that if you have an overgrowth of Candida yeast, your probiotics will not colonize your gut!

Everyday Nutritional Supplements

Changing your eating habits is essential for growing a new body and sustaining its benefits. But it can be challenging to follow all the dietary recommendations, especially at the times of the year when farm-fresh, locally grown produce isn't available in your area. Nutritional supplements can help you get on the fast track to repair your gut and maintain a brain-friendly diet.

We have spoken about many of these supplements in the previous chapter, but only in the context of the program. Here we will review them in the role they can have in your everyday diet. These supplements all play a role in how your brain and the organs in your body repair and regenerate. Be sure to check with your health-care professional before taking any supplements, and listen to your body. There's a right dosage for each person, and it's slightly different for everyone, even during different seasons. Pay close attention to how you feel, and learn your body's subtle messages.

These are the nutritional supplements you should consider taking on a regular basis:

DHA, docosahexaenoic acid, is an omega-3 fatty acid that is essential for brain health. In fact, 40 percent of the brain is made of DHA and nearly 50 percent of breast milk. DHA is found in fish, nuts, seeds, and certain oils. Since the body doesn't manufacture DHA, you need to supplement either from fish oil or algae. Researchers have noted an 85 percent reduction in the risk for Alzheimer's among people with high levels of DHA in their diet.[10] Be sure to take your DHA in the evening so that your body does not burn it as fuel and it can get to your brain to turn on the production of BDNF and neural stem cells.

We used to get our DHA from wild-caught fish, but today most of our fish is farm raised, and fed on corn, and contains very little DHA. As a result, many people's brains are unable to repair. If you notice others around you becoming duller and less able to relate, it's likely because their brains are broken from lack of DHA in their diet.

The dosage is 2 grams daily.

ALA, alpha-lipoic acid, is found in every cell in the body and plays a crucial role in detoxification. ALA will cross the blood-brain barrier, and ferry toxins, including heavy metals, out of the brain. The liver loves ALA.

The dosage is 300 to 600 mg, 3 days a week (does not need to be taken daily).

Turmeric increases levels of superoxide dismutase (SOD) and glutathione—two antioxidants important to brain functioning that are described in detail in Chapter 7, Resetting the Death Clock. Its powers include cancer prevention, elimination of free radicals, and support for the heart, liver, and gastrointestinal system. Turmeric has very poor bioavailability—that is, less than 5 percent of what you ingest actually gets into your system. Use it in curries and salads.

The dosage is 1,000 mg daily.

Vitamin B12 is essential for liver detoxification and for repairing the myelin sheath around nerves. It is also needed for preserving the integrity of DNA and for production of neurotransmitters. Most Americans are B12 deficient. Take sublingual methylcobalamin B12—a more bioavailable form.

The dosage is 2,500 mcg a day.

Vitamin C is essential for all detoxification processes.

The dosage is 1,000 mg a day.

Vitamin D3 is the form of vitamin D that the body manufactures when it's exposed to sunlight. But even if you spend a great deal time outdoors, it's unlikely you're getting enough vitamin D3. Vitamin D deficiency has been linked to seasonal depression, diabetes, dementia, and autoimmune disorders. Individuals who take 600 international units (IU) or more of vitamin D3 are half as likely to develop dementia and Alzheimer's compared to control groups.[11] Dosage varies widely, but in a review of current research, vitamin D expert Michael Holick, M.D., cites therapeutic doses for adults ranging from 1,000 IU a day to 10,000 IU a day.[12] I like to work with a dose in the middle of this range.

The dosage is 5,000 IU daily.

Coconut oil and MCT oil are jet fuel for the brain. These medium-chain triglycerides pass through the intestinal wall without causing an insulin spike and go into the mitochondria inside cells. Take two tablespoons daily—one tablespoon in the morning and one tablespoon midafternoon, together with MCT oil in the same proportion. You can also add coconut oil to soup and tea. I like to eat it straight from the jar, like ice cream!

The dosage is 4 tablespoons (1/4 cup) daily, preferably in the morning.

Ubiquinol is a more efficient version of coenzyme Q10, which is essential for energy production by our mitochondria. When mice who were fed ubiquinol during their lives reached the equivalent of 90 years of human age, they were still "going skiing" compared with a control group of mice that were riddled with cancers and heart disease.
The dosage is 200 mg daily.

Multivitamin and mineral formula is essential as even the most beautiful-looking organic vegetables you find in stores are grown on depleted soils. Get a good-quality multivitamin from a known brand and take it daily.
Take the dosage indicated in the product.

Zinc is needed by the liver to detox. The World Health Organization estimates that one in three persons is deficient in zinc.
The dosage is 15 mg daily.

Magnesium is essential for the liver to move toxins out of the bloodstream and into the GI tract for elimination. It is probably the most important mineral in the body, and most of us are magnesium deficient. Signs of deficiency include muscle aches, anxiety, and trouble sleeping.
The dosage is 350 mg daily.

New Supplements in This Edition

These supplements can help you maintain strong bones and prevent disease, as well as providing you with essential co-factors for producing cellular energy.

Vitamin K2 has not received much attention in the Western diet, and many people have not even heard of it. Vitamin K2, particularly menaquinone-7 (MK-7), keeps calcium out of your arteries and in your bones by switching on mineralization by osteoblasts (the bone-building cells). It increases bone mass and mechanical strength to produce tough but supple bone that is more resistant to fracture. The population in the United States is vitamin K deficient because we do not consume sufficient greens. In Japan, people get MK-7 from a fermented soy product called natto, which accounts for the decreased risks of fractures and bone loss among Japanese women. Vitamin K2 reduces the risk for heart disease.

The dosage is 100 mcg daily.

Sodium bicarbonate, also known as baking soda, can help you neutralize the overly acidic Western diet and reset your pH. Organic sodium bicarbonate is a great home remedy for reflux, as it neutralizes stomach acids. Be sure to wait at least two hours after your last meal to take baking soda so that you do not interfere with your digestion. Carbon dioxide is produced as stomach acids are neutralized so you may find yourself burping after taking sodium bicarbonate.

The dosage is ½ teaspoon in the evening two hours after your meal.

Nicotinamide riboside is a newly discovered natural form of vitamin B3 that when used in conjunction with pterostilbene, increases the concentrations of NAD+ in the brain by 40 percent, allowing for more efficient energy production. NAD+ levels decrease with age, and supporting them with nicotinamide riboside might offer significant protection to brain cells.

The dosage is 125 mg daily.

Tryptophan (also called L-tryprophan) is an essential amino acid that acts like a natural hormone balancer and mood regulator. Supplementing with tryptophan induces sleep, calms anxiety, and can help burn more body fat. Tryptophan will reduce carb cravings and help lower sugar addiction. Tryprophan increases the production of serotonin, the "feel good" neurotransmitter. Supplementing with tryptophan will help control appetite and make it easier to lose weight. It will also support the production of DMT inside the brain.

The dosage is 1,000 mg daily.

During the Grow a New Body program, you will be taking additional supplements described later in the book.

Nutritional supplements are powerful substances and should be used with caution. If you choose to take the supplements discussed in this book, check with a physician and nutritionist. Be sure, when choosing supplements, that you favor gelcaps over capsules and capsules over tablets, to make it easier for your gut to absorb the ingredients.

PART III

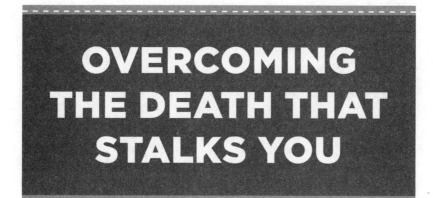

**OVERCOMING
THE DEATH THAT
STALKS YOU**

Chapter 7

RESETTING THE DEATH CLOCK

There is no greater mistake than to try to leap an abyss in two jumps.

— DAVID LLOYD GEORGE, BRITISH PRIME MINISTER

Mother Nature wants you to be "fruitful and multiply, and to fill the earth," so that humanity will not be threatened with extinction. Thus, while potential immortality belongs to the human species, death claims the individual. At around age 35, toward the end of your reproductive years, vital repair and regeneration systems in your body begin to decline. You stop producing growth hormone, which builds muscle and keeps skin youthful and elastic. Your levels of glutathione and SOD (superoxide dismutase), the free-radical scavengers, drop pretty much to zero by the time you are 40. Wrinkles appear, you do not heal as quickly as you once did, and your notion of a late night out means being in bed by 11 P.M.

Nature doesn't have many plans for you once you are over your childbearing years. I hate to say it, but biology conspires for the young. As we grow older, our body performs a kind of triage, explains Bruce Ames, Ph.D., director of the Center for Nutrition and Metabolism at Children's Hospital in Oakland, California. Essential vitamins and minerals are offered first to the proteins needed for survival, at the expense of longevity proteins like SIRT-1 that are essential for long-term health.[1]

Many of us are deficient in one or more longevity-ensuring nutrients. Among the poor, this is largely due to malnutrition. Among the affluent, who often are eating a calorie-rich but nutrient-poor diet, deficiency is usually due to malabsorption of nutrients by a gut damaged by antibiotics. The liver can store a few years' worth of vitamin B12, but if you are not able to absorb B12 from your food, you will be deficient in this essential vitamin. Almost everyone in the U.S. is magnesium and selenium deficient.

Ames uses the example of vitamin K, which the body needs for blood clotting and healthy bones. If you do not get enough of this essential vitamin from the greens in your diet, your body will perform a kind of triage and deploy the available vitamin K to produce clotting factors that will keep you from bleeding to death from a cut. There will not be enough vitamin K to remove calcium from your blood and deposit it in your bones where it is needed to prevent osteoporosis, and you will become a candidate for the perfect heart-attack storm from calcium buildup in your arteries. This is another reason why a good quality multivitamin is so important for your health.

We have all heard that youth is wasted on the young. Indigenous peoples prize adolescent beauty and feats of strength and endurance but also the wisdom of age. For them, knowledge is not held in books but in the memory of the elders. If this wisdom is lost to dementia, the entire culture is endangered. Amazon shamans discovered plants that protect the brain as we grow older, without being able to explain the science underlying what they learned. They found that certain plants eliminated the debris inside brain cells and repaired the mitochondria, the power centers in the cell, so that their elders remembered the teaching stories and songs. Like these wise elders, we can work with these plant substances to write a new chapter in our lives after age 35. Then, we are much more likely to enjoy a long health span and take our brain and memory with us into our later years.

Switching on the longevity system begins with repairing our cells' power factories: the mitochondria.

Repairing the Mitochondria

Our ancestors didn't have a clue, of course, what mitochondria were. They refer to whatever prevented aging and decline as "the feminine life force." Today, science offers us a less mystical explanation.

Mitochondria are tiny organelles inside every cell, and their main job is to convert carbohydrates and fats into energy in the process known as metabolism. Mitochondria are actually bacteria that evolved from the first oxygen-breathing organisms on Earth. Billions of years ago, early bacteria fed on amino acids and the abundant chemicals in the primordial soup of the Earth's oceans. As food supplies became scarce, the first blue-green algae appeared and discovered a new food source, the sun, and a way of using sunlight as fuel. This new discovery—photosynthesis—was a monumental breakthrough. Now there was abundant food for any organisms that could feed directly on sunlight, and blue-green algae became the most successful life-form on the planet. But green plants produce as a by-product a highly poisonous gas: oxygen. Much of the free oxygen in the atmosphere was absorbed by the rocks, but once those were saturated, oxygen levels in the atmosphere built up rapidly. Since life-forms at that time did not breathe oxygen, this resulted in a global catastrophe, an extinction event in which 99 percent of all species perished. There was an exception: mitochondria, the first and only oxygen-breathing bacteria, who now became the most successful life-form on Earth.

As life evolved, mitochondria insinuated themselves into the bodies of plants and animals, enjoying a harmonious relationship with their hosts. In exchange for a warm, safe environment, they supplied fuel to the host. Every creature, plant, and animal living today relies on mitochondria for their fuel needs.

Mitochondria have their own DNA, separate from ours, and while the structure of our DNA is a double helix, theirs, like all bacterial DNA, resembles a string of pearls (in other words, a ring). We have more than 24,000 genes; mitochondria have only 38. But oh, how important those 38 genes are! Not only are mitochondria the body's fuel factories, they are also the keepers of the death clock, controlling the process of cell death, known as apoptosis. When the death clock is running properly, old cells know exactly when they need to die to be replaced by healthy new ones. But when the death clock is off, cells don't know they need to die, and the result is cancer. Or they die off too quickly, and the result is accelerated aging.

The Fuel of Life

Mitochondrial DNA is handed down through the mother's genes, and they quite literally represent the feminine life force, passed from mother to daughter. Millions of years ago the first eukaryotic cells—those with a nucleus—thrived when they allied with mitochondria. Similarly, human bodies today can thrive if we nurture this feminine force. Mitochondria provide the fuel we need to live: ATP, or adenosine triphosphate. When we feed them ketones, particularly one called β-hydroxybutyrate, they provide the fuel to switch on the neural networks that facilitate the experience of Oneness.

Years ago I spent a few weeks at a Buddhist center in Santa Fe, New Mexico. No matter how hard I prayed or concentrated, my mind kept wandering to my to-do list, or to the attractive woman sitting in front of me. Then I decided to fast, drinking only water for four days. The first two days were awful—not only was I fidgeting on my meditation cushion, but the growling in my stomach was disturbing everyone around me. But by day three, everything changed. My hunger pangs had disappeared, and meditation came easy. The woman in front of me was not a distraction any longer, the constant chatter inside my head stopped, and I was experiencing a newfound sense of peace. All of this came with ease, without effort.

It takes two to three days to burn through the residual sugars in your bloodstream and switch to using fat for fuel. These ketones were turning on higher brain functions I had been trying to reach by sitting cross-legged on a meditation pillow. My limbic brain and its Neanderthal instincts wanted nothing to do with meditation—it wanted to spring into action slaying dragons or rescuing fair maidens or checking e-mails. That day I realized that what we call spiritual experiences are not only the result of our meditation practice, but of our brain chemistry. We need both.

Today I bring a jar of coconut oil whenever I go on a retreat and give it to all of our participants in our Grow a New Body programs to help them get over the hump of the first couple of days it takes to switch into ketosis.

It's All about the Money

ATP is the body's currency: the cells spend what they need to repair and divide and deposit the rest in the bank, the liver, where it is stored until needed to power various body functions. To produce ATP, mitochondria combust oxygen, in much the way your automobile engine burns oxygen, releasing the energy in fuel—though in a far less explosive fashion. As we inhale, the oxygen is transported by the bloodstream to our cells, where mitochondria use it to burn glucose and fats to make ATP.

Without healthy, high-functioning mitochondria, every cell is at risk. Some 200 ailments we suffer from today—from cancer, heart disease, fibromyalgia, and chronic fatigue to Parkinson's disease, dementia, cirrhosis of the liver, and migraine headaches—have been linked to mitochondrial dysfunction. Mitochondria are easily damaged by toxins, including pharmaceuticals. Reviewing current research, naturopath John Neustadt and psychiatrist Steve Pieczenik found that "medications have now emerged as a major cause of mitochondrial damage, which may explain many adverse effects. All classes of psychotropic drugs have been documented to damage mitochondria, as have statin medications, analgesics such as acetaminophen, and many others."[2]

Damaged mitochondria reproduce more quickly than healthy ones and feed on sugars, unlike healthy mitochondria, which can also feed on fats. Because cancer cells, with their deficient mitochondria, burn glucose as their primary fuel, researchers believe that reducing or eliminating sugar-rich carbs is an effective means of fighting and preventing cancer.[3]

When mitochondria are damaged, your metabolism becomes sluggish. You have no energy. Your body no longer remembers how to burn fat, and you can't lose weight. The fat stores in your body become repositories for toxins. You're likely to feel moody, fatigued, and generally unwell. With big dips in energy, you're more likely to reach for a quick fix like a sugary protein bar, which only exacerbates the problem by feeding the sugar-hungry yeast in your gut and raising your blood-glucose levels. Inflammation results, oxidative stress worsens, and more mitochondria are damaged.

Defective mitochondria accumulate inside the cells, accelerating aging, and damaged cells grow uncontrollably, forming tumors.

Autophagy, or Recycling Mitochondria

Eliminating broken and ailing mitochondria and supporting the birth of vibrant, potent mitochondria are crucial for brain repair. As we learned earlier, autophagy is the garbage disposal service inside the cells, the process by which cellular waste is broken down and damaged mitochondria are recycled to harvest amino acids, the building blocks of new cells. So just as dead plants in the forest get turned into food for new plants with the help of microbes that break them down, your body has a system for recycling the amino acids from dead and damaged mitochondria to make new cells. It is called autophagy.

Aerobic exercise triggers autophagy: exercise consumes oxygen, which starves off the weakest mitochondria while fostering the growth of more vigorous ones. Detoxifying is another way to jump-start mitochondria. And eating a diet high in phytonutrients switches on the antioxidant production inside the cell that repairs mitochondria and supports autophagy. But ultimately, the master switch of autophagy is mTOR.

The most effective way of supporting autophagy is through fasting. Even a short 18-hour fast between dinner and lunch the next day causes the body to go into repair mode, as mTOR sensors register the drop in nutrients. The body's ability to switch over to burning fat gave us an edge when it came to surviving harsh winters when food was scarce. But our mitochondria can't make the switch if our fat deposits become waste dumps for toxins. The body in its wisdom will not burn fats if they are full of poison. To switch from carb-burning to fat-burning, you have to begin recycling waste and eliminating toxins.

Consuming healthy fats like avocados, coconut oil, and olive oil fuels the brain and the heart (and all our mitochondria) with ketone bodies, which are many times more efficient a fuel than sugars.[4] But as soon as you reach for carbs, the mitochondria treat the sugar as the first course, filling up and forgetting about the rest of the meal. The extra sugar has to go somewhere, so your pancreas produces insulin to transport it to cells that can use it. But if the cells already have plenty of glucose on board, they'll refuse the delivery, just as if they were pushing away a dessert plate. Since there's no point in letting that delicious chocolate cake go to waste, your body will make sure the glucose is stored as fat.

When high blood sugar becomes chronic, you have a prediabetic condition. Unable to absorb more sugar, your cells reduce the number of insulin receptors. But the pancreas, registering a buildup of sugar levels in your blood, continues to pump out more insulin. The result is insulin resistance.

If you're consuming large amounts of carbs, gaining weight around your belly, and experiencing mood swings and brain fog, you're already on your way toward insulin resistance and mitochondrial damage. By changing to a diet high in plant foods and healthy fats and low in carbs, your pancreas will quiet the insulin system that activates the mTOR pathway. Autophagy will kick in. Toxins stored inside cells will be eliminated. Dead mitochondria will be recycled for their amino acids. The system will run as it's supposed to.

Reducing Oxidative Stress and Free-Radical Activity

Mitochondria combust oxygen to produce energy. But like that old car of yours that burned oil and released clouds of black smoke from the exhaust, when metabolism isn't efficient—when it doesn't burn clean—it produces hazardous free radicals. And mitochondria are easily damaged by free radicals. Damaged mitochondria produce more free radicals. And the free radicals damage fats, proteins, and even the DNA in our cell nuclei.

Environmental toxins worsen the situation. Most dangerous are pesticides, which work by destroying the mitochondria of invasive pests and are designed to stick to the plants and not wash off easily in the rain, or when you rinse your vegetables at home. And residual pesticides have the same deadly effect on your mitochondria as they do on pests.

The more oxidative stress on your body, the more antioxidants you will need. You can get antioxidants from foods like berries, but you would need to eat close to 40 pounds of blueberries a day to neutralize the billions of free radicals circulating through your body. Fortunately, the body can produce natural antioxidants like glutathione and SOD. Unfortunately, these endogenous antioxidants stop being produced around the age of 35, and their levels drop down to zero by the time you are 40 years old.

An amazing discovery of the shamans were the medicinal plants that could switch back on the dormant antioxidant systems. Nrf2 activators like trans-resveratrol curcumin and pterostilbene restore the free-radical scavengers to the levels you enjoyed in your 20s. And we will learn how you can do this in as little as seven days.

Inflammation

Localized inflammation is a natural and healthy immune response. When you fall and hurt your knee, white blood cells rush to the area to trap foreign matter like bacteria so they can be neutralized. But chronic inflammation disturbs the body's equilibrium, and the immune system will begin to attack healthy cells and tissues, mistaking them for foreign invaders. The death clock speeds up when inflammation goes unchecked, and you develop heart disease and autoimmune disorders like rheumatoid arthritis, diabetes, and multiple sclerosis.

Chronic inflammation can damage brain structures, including the hippocampus, and can lead to conditions like Parkinson's disease and Alzheimer's. Fortunately, the Nrf2 activators at the core of the Grow a New Body program have extraordinary anti-inflammatory properties. Researchers have discovered that even common anti-inflammatory medications like aspirin and ibuprofen will lower Alzheimer's risk by as much as 60 percent[5] and reduce the risk of Parkinson's disease by a staggering 45 percent![6]

Repairing the Hippocampus

Shaped like a sea horse, the hippocampus helps us to regulate our emotions as well as to store memories and learn. Any new skill, from playing a musical instrument to learning to eat for health and longevity, requires the participation of the hippocampus. So when the hippocampus is damaged, curiosity and enthusiasm for life drift away. We are left angry or afraid. Repairing it with omega-3 fish oils, however, can help heal our emotions and with memory and learning.

Damage to the hippocampus can impair short-term memory while leaving long-term memory intact. That may help explain why often people with dementia can recall events from many years in the past yet are unable to remember what happened two weeks or even ten minutes ago.

The hippocampus cannot tell time, so it often confuses something happening today with something similar that happened 20 years ago. That new person we just met may trigger memories of a former lover from years back, and that's where the conversation ends. And the hippocampus is linked not just to past events but also to old behaviors, worn-out thoughts, and used-up feelings. When it's damaged, we keep recalling the same painful situations, the same painful emotions, over and over again. We aren't as open to new experiences and learning.

A few years back, a friend invited me to his wedding—his fifth. When I reminded him of this, he told me that this time was different. My friend was trying to repair his hippocampus, and have a new experience, through yet another marriage—not a very practical way to go about repairing the brain. I suggested to him that he stop looking for the right partner and start working on *becoming* the right partner. He was not very happy with my advice. Six months after the wedding he called and told me his marriage was over—and he was angry with me that I allowed him to marry such a cruel and thoughtless person. I reminded him of what the scholar and mythologist Joseph Campbell once said—if you don't learn a lesson, you end up marrying it. I told my friend that unless he repaired his hippocampus, most likely he would keep seeking—and finding—the same kind of partner again, with a different name.

My friend's repetitious behavior was distracting him from opening his eyes to what is new—to the opportunities for new experiences. Time was ticking away. Yet he was still looking for love in the same old way. By using the Grow a New Body protocol, you can grow a new brain that is not stuck in the past, responding instead with fresh insights and approaches, and falling in love for all the right reasons.

When our hippocampus is damaged, we perceive everything around us as a threatening situation. When the hippocampus is healed, we begin to see opportunity where we once saw only crisis. I have a patient, for instance, who has made a fortune in the stock market investing in companies that everyone else was selling at a time of perceived danger.

You heal the hippocampus by increasing your level of serotonin (made by the flora in your gut) and switching on the production of stem cells in the brain. A couple of decades ago we believed that the brain was not able to grow new neurons. Today we know that the brain can produce new stem cells and repair in as little as six weeks, knitting new neural networks as you learn fresh ways of looking at life. You can change your life by changing your brain, instead of by replacing your spouse, getting a new job, or shipping your kids off to boarding school. That is easier to do when you have a robust hippocampus to help you.

Just as updating the operating system on your computer lets you run new, more powerful programs and applications, upgrading the learning centers in your brain sets you up for new, more creative thinking that can enhance your health and emotional well-being.

When you become forgetful, you may be tempted to laugh off the befuddlement as a "senior moment," while secretly harboring fear of Alzheimer's and dementia. The idea that the mind is deteriorating with age is terrifying, but aging does not have to include loss of brain function. The illnesses characteristic of aging in the West, including cardiovascular disease, Alzheimer's, dementia, and Parkinson's, are largely preventable. Prevention starts with growing new brain cells in the hippocampus, along with eating a diet that will fuel your brain with good fats.

Boosting Brain Health with BDNF, Glutathione, and SOD

Our Paleolithic ancestors may have known little about brain chemistry, but they were savvy about the plants that could switch on the brain's ability to upgrade itself. Now scientists have discovered three key substances that repair the brain. Even more amazing is that these three products turn on your ability to produce neural stem cells and can actually help you grow a new and healthier brain.

BDNF, brain-derived neurotrophic factor, stimulates the development of new brain cells and is vital for repairing and rewiring the brain so that new ways of thinking, perceiving, and responding will emerge spontaneously. When was the last time you fell in love all over again with your partner or spouse? BDNF updates your brain so you can experience the re-enchantment of your life and your world.

How important is BDNF? Inadequate BDNF production is associated with Alzheimer's, dementia, and depression. Toxins, stress, lack of exercise, and a sugary diet all lower BDNF levels. If you're not getting enough omega-3s from foods, then supplementing with omega-3 fatty acids is essential to increase BDNF levels and to upgrade your brain.

How to increase it: Fasting overnight and then breaking the fast with fats like an avocado rather than carbs will increase your BDNF. But to boost it further, you might consider doing a one-day water-only fast during the seven-day Grow a New Body program. Exercise is another way to increase BDNF levels, but make sure you choose a form of exercise you enjoy: research shows that exercise you like is better for generating BDNF than something you do only because you know you ought to.

Glutathione is an antioxidant and anti-inflammatory. It neutralizes free radicals, and as a detoxifying agent, it serves as a sort of lint brush, picking up toxins in the body and carrying them to the liver for processing. Glutathione boosts your immunity and helps you build and maintain muscle. Low glutathione levels increase free-radical damage to your mitochondria, which then are unable to regulate the cells' death clocks.

How to increase it: Foods like kale, spinach, avocado, and squash increase the body's ability to produce glutathione. However, many people, including me, lack the GSTM1 gene, which is necessary for manufacturing glutathione, and nearly half the world is missing one or more of the genes necessary to produce glutathione. Among the critically ill, the percentage is even higher: a majority of people with chronic disease have negligible glutathione levels.

Because the body can't utilize glutathione in regular supplement form—it's easily destroyed in the gut—I recommend the oral form of S-acetyl glutathione, which can make it through the gut and into the bloodstream. You will take 1,000 mg daily S-acetyl glutathione during the Grow a New Body program.

You can also take NAC (N-acetylcysteine), which helps boost production of glutathione. The benefit of taking NAC over s-acetyl glutathione is that the body can use this precursor to glutathione to manufacture glutathione at its own rate when needed, rather than receiving a high dose taken all at once.

SOD, or superoxide dismutase, is the ultimate antioxidant, an enzyme that neutralizes free radicals in a ratio of over a million to one—in other words, one molecule of SOD kills one million free radicals. Vitamins C and E are also considered great antioxidants, but they have a kill ratio of only one to one. Since there are zillions of free radicals in the body—far too many for one little vitamin pill to quench—we need the firepower of SOD to effectively reduce damaging oxidative stress.

Low levels of SOD play a role in atherosclerosis—hardening of the arteries associated with aging—and in collagen breakdown in aging skin. Our bodies produce SOD naturally, and it can also be found in foods, but reversing a lifetime of free-radical onslaught from exposure to pesticides and environmental toxins requires a major intervention.

How to increase it: You can upgrade your body's ability to manufacture SOD by taking the supplements trans-resveratrol (500 mg daily) and curcumin (1,000 mg daily). You can also boost SOD by adding pterostilbene-rich foods to your diet—eating more blueberries and grapes, for example—or by taking a pterostilbene supplement.

While increasing BDNF, glutathione, and SOD can repair your mitochondria and prevent the ravages of the diseases of old age, they are also important for another reason: They clear the debris in the brain and allow us to experience Oneness. The experience of Oneness allows you to create health and dream your world into being in a powerful and creative way.

Chapter 8

FREEING YOURSELF FROM STRESSORS

The major advances in civilization are processes which all but wreck the societies in which they occur.

— Alfred North Whitehead, British mathematician and philosopher

Years ago, my mentor among the Amazon shamans told me that to learn the wisdom of the rain forest, I would have to spend a night alone in the jungle along a tributary of the Mother of God River. He left me off at a distant beach just as the sun was setting. It was a beautiful spot—a white sandy clearing surrounded by gigantic trees known as *shihuahuacos*. Across the river, parrots and macaws were feasting on a natural clay lick, nibbling on the red earth to ingest the minerals that are part of their morning and evening meals. The setting sun cast its ocher rays on the face of the clay lick, making the blue and red feathers of the birds seem translucent. And then suddenly, as happens in the jungle in the tropics, it was dark.

I rummaged through my pack and discovered that the old man had taken my flashlight and the matches I always carried for such an occasion. I tried to talk myself into believing that I was in Eden, that there was much beauty all around me, and that I was safe. Yet as night descended, the full shock of being alone in the dark jungle hit me, and I was terrified. Every snap of a twig or rustling of leaves alarmed me. I was certain I was being stalked by a jaguar that would pounce any second and sink its teeth into me. And then the morning arrived and everything seemed fine again, even after I saw the fresh jaguar tracks in the sand. It wasn't until I had spent much more time in the rain forest that I understood that I could be safe there even with minimal provisions. I learned not to be prey for jaguars.

We become prey for jaguars and others who would devour us when they smell our fear. A jaguar can track your scent from miles away, just as a mugger in the inner city can pick you out as his target with an uncanny sense of knowing which people are easy marks. Fear launches a chemical cascade in your brain and hormonal system that literally changes your scent to that of a hunted animal. Have you even been so afraid that you could smell the fear in your own sweat? Then your mind casts the world as predatory, and you focus on self-protection: *Am I safe? Do I have enough love or money or whatever else I need to feel secure?* Fear keeps you in a chronic hyperalert state that can turn you into someone's dinner.

Our fear can make us sick. Many of the health problems we face are caused by our unhealed emotions, and paramount among these is fear. Emotions are ancient survival programs encoded in the limbic brain, and when toxic emotions dominate your thinking and nervous system, you put yourself in danger. To stop being the victim of your circumstances and become a hero embarking on an epic journey of discovery, you will need to heal your emotions. You won't have to go out of your way to find opportunities to heal. Life presents plenty of challenges and stressors that will allow you to transform toxic emotions like fear and anger into positive feelings like compassion and love.

I like to distinguish between toxic emotions, which can fester and poison us, and feelings, which are authentic, of the moment, and transitory. You might have an occasional feeling of anger toward your children or spouse, a spontaneous flash that sends a surge of chemicals through your body and brain, but the feeling soon passes and equanimity returns. Toxic emotions, on the other hand, can linger in the body and take up residence in neural networks in the brain for hours or days or years. The brain scientist Jill Bolte Taylor describes the difference between feeling and emotion in *My Stroke of Insight: A Brain Scientist's Personal Journey*: "Within 90 seconds from the initial trigger, the chemical component of my anger has completely dissipated from my blood and my automatic response is over. If, however, I remain angry after those 90 seconds have passed, then it is because I have *chosen* to let that circuit continue to run. Moment by moment, I make the choice to either hook into my neurocircuitry or move back into the present moment."[1]

Fear is one of the deadliest emotions. It blinds us to opportunities around us. Terror sees no way out. Fear triggers the fight-or-flight system, known as the HPA axis, which consists of the hypothalamus and the pituitary gland, pea-sized structures in the brain, and the adrenal glands, which sit atop the kidneys. When you sense danger, perceived or real, the brain launches a distress response in the HPA axis, reducing the blood flow to your prefrontal cortex, the part of the brain that can sense opportunities.

There are real dangers in the world. But you have a choice about how you respond to them. To stop being prey, you need to let go of beliefs that reinforce your view of the world as predatory. Once you understand that it is your beliefs that cause stress and not people or situations "out there," you will be able to live in harmony with the world around you instead of feeling as if you're trapped forever in a combat zone.

The emotional pressure we experience in everyday life is often the result of our limiting beliefs and an overactive fight-or-flight response.

Limiting Beliefs

Limiting beliefs have nothing to do with IQ or education and everything to do with early life experiences that shape our worldview, which the brain's ever-efficient yet unconscious neural networks interpret as reality. It sometimes seems as if the more knowledgeable experts are, the more likely they are to be blinded by their beliefs. Before the U.S. invaded Iraq, countless experts testified that Saddam Hussein was stockpiling weapons of mass destruction; later, of course, none was found. The "facts" presented to the American people were bogus. The experts who testified before Congress were not lying; they were simply convinced they had a lock on the truth. Have you seen the magazine advertisements from the 1950s that say, "More doctors smoke Camels than any other cigarette"?

In forming an opinion, we give weight to facts that fit with our beliefs and readily dismiss those that don't. Take fake news, for example. While two friends can agree that much of the news we read is fake, they will completely disagree as to which news is real. Western society favors science and reason over intuition, seldom blending the two different ways of knowing to gain a broader perspective. When I talk to people who have a medical background, they always want to know the scientific research that supports my statements about health, even when they instinctively know what I'm saying is true. That's one reason I've included so much science in a book: we want to see research papers published in professional journals that validate age-old advice. And even when it comes to science, a lot of what is published in journals and passed off as serious science is also fake. Sometimes scientists retrofit their hypotheses to fit their data, or base conclusions on studies with sample sizes that are too small or produce miniscule effects.[2]

The more we rely exclusively on one way of knowing, however, the more likely we are to operate from biases we aren't even aware of. Our insistence on valuing science over intuition ignores findings that when we combine the two, we often make better decisions. Researchers Douglas Dean and John Mihalasky did a ten-year study of ESP (extrasensory perception, that is, intuition) in business executives. They found that CEOs who trusted intuition and took risks based on their hunches made significantly more money than CEOs who made decisions based solely on logic and "facts."[3]

Intuition isn't necessarily as irrational as hardcore rationalists assume. Nobel prizewinners Herbert Simon and Daniel Kahneman are among those whose research has found that when experts make decisions based on intuition, they're actually drawing on a storehouse of experience and knowledge.[4] By contrast, a decision made on a hunch like *I don't know why I chose him; I just liked his look* is more likely a purely emotional response and has as much chance of being wrong as being right. I am convinced that much of what we call intuition is really a gut instinct that is available to us all once we repair our gut and upgrade the colony of good bacteria that make up more than 90 percent of who we are.

A common bias that can have grave consequences is the belief that we aren't equipped to protect our own health but must rely on doctors, drugs, and therapies to heal us. This leads to a feeling of powerlessness that can prevent us from taking lifesaving action on our own behalf. The Grow a New Brain program will help you recognize that you don't need to depend on medical experts or drugs alone. You can draw on the power of superfoods and neuronutrients, combined with the resources of Spirit to support your innate self-healing ability.

As long as we're caught in the grip of our limiting beliefs stored in the limbic brain, we will constantly look to others to tell us what to do—not just medical experts to determine our health care but also political commentators to tell us how to vote and the media to show us who our enemies are.

Our limiting beliefs tend to keep us trapped in one of three roles: victim, persecutor, or rescuer. These sit at the three corners of what I call the triangle of disempowerment. We create dramas featuring these stock roles, and then as the story unfolds, we act as if lost in a maze. We never break out of the disempowering tale, holding on with a death grip to the parts we are playing or simply switching roles, which keeps us trapped in the triangle. Small wonder every situation seems familiar: we keep projecting the same stories onto the players and reenacting the old dramas.

New patients who come to see me for energy medicine often want me to be the rescuer who heals them from whatever ailment is keeping them a victim. My first task is to refuse that job and instead help my patients find their own inner resources to heal. Otherwise, they will expect me to perform magic while they remain passive observers.

All these roles—victim, persecutor, rescuer—keep us feeling scared, defensive, envious, and competitive. When we encounter someone who is doing something clever or original, instead of admiring that person, we feel jealous, or we belittle their efforts. As writer Gore Vidal is credited with saying, "Every time a friend of mine succeeds, a little part of me dies." The opportunity we face is to move beyond our limiting beliefs and understand our lives in a larger context, unfettered by biases that distort our perceptions. Heroic narratives about people who have been tested and then overcome their wounds to heal themselves are far more empowering than the three-character dramas we habitually create. They can inspire us instead of locking us into a story about how unfair our lives are.

To change our inner narratives, we have to repair our fight-or-flight system. Once you reset the HPA axis, you can more readily choose to release negative emotions that feed depression, anger, and that make you sick, and cultivate positive feelings that help the body repair.

Overstimulation and Fight-or-Flight

Two stressors we face today—overstimulation and an overactive fight-or-flight system—often go hand in hand. We're bombarded with more information and sensory stimulation than we can possibly handle, which sets off our HPA axis.

From television and the Internet, we're exposed to more stimuli in a week than our Paleolithic ancestors were exposed to in a lifetime. And we're continually running to keep up with new information, to the point that we're chronically exhausted. I can't count how many times I have heard someone say, "If it weren't for caffeine, I wouldn't get anything done!" Nature designed the brain to deal with only one lion roaring at us at a time, not the entire jungle turning against us. Now, however, our brain is too overtaxed to sort through all the data, much less look at it with fresh eyes and decide what is or is not a crisis, and what, if anything, needs to be done about it.

The media bring us news about wars happening in distant lands, but our fight-or-flight response operates only with local coordinates and doesn't understand *far away*. When we read about some catastrophic event, the higher brain grasps that it's happening at another time and place. But when the lower limbic brain, which regulates the fight-or-flight response, is presented with streaming video of an atrocity, it registers it as happening *now* and *nearby* and goes on high alert. The more damaged by stress and toxins our hippocampus, the closer and more threatening the danger appears to be, until it seems to be right outside the village gates or your own apartment.

Although it isn't often talked about, the fight-or-flight system actually has a "freeze" element. When you perceive danger, you might get angry and scared and put up a fight, or you might run away, but you also can become paralyzed. Often, we freeze in response to the incoming information, becoming very slow to react. This is because our feelings are conveyed by hormones traveling through the body in a slow chemical system you can think of as analog, not digital. We're operating on old technology.

We are an analog creature in today's digital world, and we cannot keep up. We are slow to shake off our feelings once they do arise in response to a situation. You can bask in the feeling of love toward a child or a pet, or seethe in anger for days. Thoughts, on the other hand, course through the nervous system at the speed of light, in digital electrical signals demanding an immediate response. Therefore, in our information-overloaded society, there is an ever-widening gap between our thoughts and our feelings, our heads and our gut. Overstimulation is the result. We sleep but do not rest. We are chronically exhausted and overworked. And this stress keeps our fight-or-flight stuck in the *on* position, poisoning the brain with stress hormones that leave us frozen in fear or felled by chronic exhaustion.

In the West we're clever at managing information overload by specializing. A physician may know about the gastrointestinal tract in exhaustive detail but be clueless when it comes to human emotions and how a patient's "gut" feeling that she is in a bad marriage might affect her physical health. Psychologists treating patients for depression or anxiety almost never think to ask about gastrointestinal problems, even though many mood disorders originate in the gut. We practice medicine by geography, with doctors specializing in hearts or brains or bones or colons but seldom putting it all together into a holistic view of the patient's wellness.

You've probably heard the expression "Neurons that fire together wire together." For many people today, the neural pathways in the brain for fight-or-flight have widened into superhighways. According to the National Institutes of Mental Health, in any given year some 25 percent of Americans qualify for a mental health diagnosis, and of those, 18 percent have anxiety and 7 percent depression.[5] Sadly, among teenagers, anxiety and depression are five to eight times as prevalent today as they were 50 years ago.[6]

The hippocampus is, in effect, the thermostat of the fight-or-flight response. It sets the threshold for what we consider danger, what we see as opportunity, and what we dismiss as irrelevant. The lower the thermostat, the less likely we are to feel spooked and the less dangerous our world seems. But when the thermostat is set high, it takes very little heat to trigger the fight-or-flight mechanism. On constant alert, we perceive danger everywhere.

And the HPA axis doesn't just control our responses to danger; it's also involved in regulating digestion, mood, sexuality, energy storage, and the immune system—which makes altering it all the more life threatening. When our fight-or-flight response is engaged, it produces adrenaline and cortisol, powerful steroid hormones. We can actually become addicted to fear and over-stimulation—or more precisely, to the chemicals they induce. It's easy to mistake a rush of adrenaline for vitality. The difference is that vitality is rejuvenating, whereas stress chemicals flooding the system lead to burnout and damage our tissues and organs, including the brain.

Addicted to Adrenaline

The hippocampus is rich in cortisol receptors; and when stress floods the system with cortisol those stress hormones damage the hippocampus, which can shrink by nearly 50 percent in size. But by nourishing the brain with omega-3 fatty acids, you can repair the hippocampus and reset the HPA axis. In as little as six weeks of supplementing with 2 grams (2,000 mg) daily of DHA, you can begin to see beauty where you saw only ugliness and sense opportunity where you perceived only danger. The hippocampus repairs quickly, and when you stop feeding your brain adrenaline and caffeine, you start to transform the negative effects of stress.

When the HPA axis is quiet, the alchemical laboratory in the pineal gland begins to produce bliss molecules that flood the brain, creating states of joy and communion. The brain cannot manufacture the chemicals for fear and stress and produce the molecules for bliss and joy at the same time. It's either one or the other.

I have a patient who was a terrible lover—at least, that's what his wife claimed. She said that for him, sex was like a deep hunger that he tried to satisfy with fast food; then, after climaxing, he would roll over and go to sleep. He focused only on the orgasm, missing the shared pleasures of foreplay. His drive to be the first to the finish line, which served him so well in his work as an investment banker, made him a loser in bed. He was unable to slow down and appreciate the intimacy. The couple came to see me after six months of unsuccessful marital therapy, and the first thing I did was put them both on a clinical dose of omega-3s of three to five grams a day (versus the maintenance dose of two grams a day). With the DHA on board and some coaching from his wife, in six weeks (which is how long it takes to upgrade the hippocampus), the man was able to discover the prize of sensual exploration. Once he reset his HPA axis, he was able to explore intimacy with his beloved.

The couple shared with several of their close friends that I was the best marital therapist they had ever been to, and a few couples wanted to see me for help with their relationships. I had to explain that I did not do talking therapy or marriage counseling, I do brain repair therapy!

When we let go of the adrenaline addiction that keeps us fired up and ready for battle, we can live more wisely. The hasty decisions and fear-driven actions we later regret happen less frequently when the HPA axis is not running the show. It's only when the brain is stuck in fight-or-flight mode that we default to clichéd, unproductive, even destructive ways, and become caught in the triangle of disempowerment.

With the bliss molecules on board, we can begin to dream again—not just at night but also during the day. Creative daydreaming is a hallmark of higher brain function. Hunter-gatherers invest only about three hours a day in procuring food and devote the rest of their time to leisure, art, and dreaming. The Hadza of Tanzania, like the !Kung of Botswana, work only about 14 hours a week. But once our forebears started farming, the amount of time devoted to ensuring they had enough food on their plates increased so much there was almost no time for sitting around the fire and exchanging stories. Industrialization was no help: time became even scarcer as workers slaved long hours in factories. It was only the people near the top or the bottom of the hierarchies of power—the superrich or the indigent monks—who were able to devote themselves to contemplation. Even now, it's difficult to meditate and daydream creatively when your days are eaten up by text messages, e-mails, and laundry.

But the importance of daydreaming cannot be overestimated. James H. Simons, a math genius of breathtaking accomplishment who started a hedge fund that made him a billionaire and a major donor to scientific causes, attributes his success to "pondering." "I wasn't the fastest guy in the world," he told *The New York Times*. "But I like to ponder. And pondering things, just sort of thinking about [them] turns out to be a pretty good approach."[7]

Gazing at the stars and imagining what might be has largely been replaced by working through an endless to-do list. Dreaming and just *being* have been pushed aside in the name of *doing*. We stand outdoors glued to our smartphones, scrolling through social media feeds, responding to text-message alerts, and checking the temperature on our weather apps instead of feeling the sun and the wind on our skin.

Technology gives us access to plenty of information. As long as we're close to a wireless hot spot, any point of contention can be settled instantly by pulling out a digital device and doing a search. What we lack is the capacity to tame all that information and experience true wisdom. Information compels us to take action—to buy, sell, perform. Wisdom compels us to dream.

Fear of Death

Limiting beliefs, overstimulation, an overactive fight-or-flight response—the mental and emotional stressors we experience all lead to our most primal fear of all: fear of death. In aboriginal societies there are rites of passage and initiations carefully designed to bring a person to directly confront the terror of death. The idea is that in experiencing death ritually, you overcome fear of that ultimate, inevitable loss. The shamans call it "living through your death," and it awakens deep wisdom about non-ordinary reality, the continuity of life in the unseen world. After that you are no longer plagued by a chronic sense of anxiety about everyday matters and can hold a larger vision of your purpose in life.

We all have a taste of this when a loved one passes. We recognize what is truly important in life, and make vows to ourselves to do more of it and less of our busy work. And then a few days or weeks later we forget, and are back at the everyday grind.

As your brain is upgraded, you will discover that you can let go of your fixation on what you think is absolutely vital to your safety and happiness and essential for your survival. As you release your old, fear-based approach to life, you will find you have more faith in your ability to handle uncertainty. You will gain a sense of living in a world that is safe and welcoming, and a universe that supports your intentions and what you value as truly important.

Separation versus Unity

The limbic brain perceives duality and separation rather than unity. It breaks reality into bite-size pieces in order to understand it, but in doing so, it misses the whole. By contrast, the higher brain senses that the visible world of matter and physical phenomena and the invisible world of Spirit and energy are not separate. It perceives the whole and not only the parts. It is only our practical, everyday perception that draws a distinction between the two. In the visible world, I perceive that my body is separate from the body of the person sitting in the chair next to me. But in the invisible world, everything is interwoven, indivisible.

The invisible world is unified, nonlocal, and beyond space-time. Though omnipresent, it is invisible to ordinary perception: we know it only through its manifestations. We can directly apprehend the invisible realm only when our perception shifts, and the barrier between the two worlds momentarily drops away. This will happen naturally and by itself as you upgrade your brain. The perception of unity and Oneness is inevitable.

Until you glimpse non-ordinary, invisible reality, your brain will remain biased toward doubting "what's out there." When you experience Oneness, the sense of separation dissolves, as you perceive yourself to be an inextricable part of the larger whole.

In the ordinary, visible world, our possibilities are limited by the information our senses can grasp. Our minds are trained to match up what we encounter today with what we've experienced in the past. But in the non-ordinary world, you can discover the origin of all things, and access a power unlimited in its potential for giving birth to the new. Seeming impossibilities become possible.

Then you can dream health and wellness into being, envision freedom from scarcity and fear, and picture harmonious interactions with other people, other creatures, and the planet. You discover that death is not something to be feared and avoided at any cost, but merely a doorway to another realm.

It was the wisdom of the invisible world that fueled the courage of ancient people to sail toward a distant horizon and settle Australia and the Pacific Islands 50,000 years ago—and to set out on foot toward the unknown and cross the Bering Strait into North America. When you draw on the wisdom of the non-ordinary realm, you can conceive of a world of endless possibility and help shape a future that hasn't gotten around to revealing itself.

The big ideas, the ones that are in synch with who we can be as opposed to who we think we ought to be, come from the non-ordinary realm. They may sound batty to people who are identified with the ordinary world and its limitations, but the energy of these ideas is too powerful, too compelling to ignore.

If you have the courage, the Grow a New Body program can pull you into an entirely different life, one with new health, new wisdom, new activities, new relationships, new opportunities. You'll begin to feel more at home in your own skin. Changes you make will stick instead of just being dreams that never become reality, and you will greet uncertainty as a familiar friend that brings you surprising opportunities.

PART IV

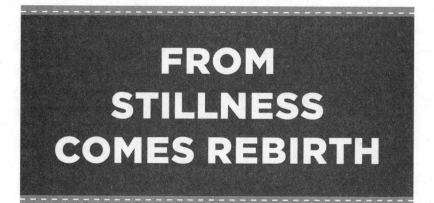

FROM
STILLNESS
COMES REBIRTH

Chapter 9

EMBRACING A NEW MYTHOLOGY

Religions, philosophies, arts, the social forms of primitive and historic man, prime discoveries in science and technology, the very dreams that blister sleep, boil up from the basic, magic ring of myth.

— Joseph Campbell, scholar and mythologist

First you eliminate the poisons in your body and upgrade your brain with superfoods and neuronutrients, switching on the genes for health and turning off the genes for disease. Then you transform your toxic emotions, reset fight-or-flight, and turn on the production of the bliss-creating molecules in your brain. The next step will be to let go of the familial and cultural myths that script your life. You can then adopt a new, more empowering myth that supports your ability to dream a new body and a new world into being.

Why mythology? Because the right side of the brain thrives on stories and myths, not facts. The success of TV series like *Game of Thrones*, films like *The Lord of the Rings* and *Star Wars*, and the Harry Potter books attest to our fascination with fantasy and myth. At the same time we tend to dismiss our popular myths as charming fables or entertaining tales. But as the scholar Joseph Campbell made clear, myths aren't just plotlines for comic books and summer blockbuster movies. They affect us to a far greater degree and at a far deeper level than we realize. From a very young age, we fall under the spell of powerful myths that influence the way we perceive the world and, consequently, the choices we make every day.

Mythologies represent the beliefs and values of particular cultures. However, certain myths seem to be universal, etched on the collective human psyche and conveying archetypal forces that crosscut time and geography. The most enduring myths involve ordinary people embarking on heroic quests, often against their will, and overcoming apparently insurmountable obstacles to perform extraordinary deeds, from the biblical Jonah who was swallowed by a whale to Luke Skywalker.

The myths of the ancient Greeks centered on the all-too-human antics of the gods on Mount Olympus and the exploits of heroes like Odysseus, Hercules, and Achilles. Our modern myths are no less compelling than those of the ancient Greeks and Romans. A classic American myth is the rags-to-riches tale of the self-made man who rises to fame and fortune through determination and hard work. Hand in hand with that is the myth of the plucky orphan who overcomes a challenging and loveless childhood thanks to her courage, dignity, and winsome charm. Like all good myths, these stories end in triumph, with virtue rewarded. Narratives like these fueled the entrepreneurial aspirations of Americans right through the end of the 20th century, when a new breed of stock trader and Internet wunderkind amassed billions overnight.

The mythic tales of the 21st century point to a different set of values. Now our myths are set in faraway star systems or magical lands inhabited by wizards and otherworldly beings. Or they reflect the shadow side of fantasy—dark, apocalyptic visions of devastation brought on by the dawn of sentient machines. Either way, we're no longer in thrall to Horatio Alger and Little

Orphan Annie. But the underlying theme remains the same: an ordinary person is called to face extraordinary challenges and is transformed in the process.

The values and beliefs contained in myths are so strong that once you find your personal guiding myth, you feel compelled to change your life to conform to it. Transform the myth and your values and beliefs are transformed—and the facts of your life change accordingly.

But you can only find your guiding myth after you've upgraded your brain because a broken brain automatically defaults to the old myths, leaving you at the mercy of the four ancient programs of the limbic brain: fighting, fleeing, feeding, and fornicating, and their corresponding myths of the warrior; the damsel in distress; the needy child; and the misguided lover. When we're caught up in aggression, fear, or greed—or its opposite, scarcity—we're unable to adopt new values and beliefs, even in the face of a serious crisis. Unconscious myths override our best intentions.

The Judeo-Christian traditions have left us with powerful myths that operate in the psyche like computer programs running continually in the background. We're not even aware of them, but they drive our basic sense of self-worth and our vision of the world, coloring the way we live from day to day.

One of the first Bible stories we learn as children is that of Adam and Eve in the book of Genesis. The myth of Adam and Eve tells us that because we disobeyed God, we're banished forever from the Garden of Eden and can no longer commune directly with God—or with the rivers and rocks and trees and animals. But indigenous people, whether sub-Saharan Africans or Australian Aborigines or Native Americans, hold no such belief about expulsion from paradise. In their mythologies, they were *not* kicked out of the Garden. In fact, they were given the Garden and entrusted with maintaining it, as the caretakers of Earth.

We may say we want to live more sustainably, in harmony with the natural world, but our old, ingrained mythic system continually hijacks our goal. We rationalize that as individuals we can't make a difference, or that the world economy would collapse if we limit emissions of greenhouse gasses. So we end up pursuing short-term economic gain and do nothing about reversing climate change. Meanwhile we walk around as creatures banished from Eden, disconnected from nature and from our divine selves.

Our Judeo-Christian tradition has given us a number of other myths, not least the idea that eternal life is for only the chosen few—and that the priests hold our passports to heaven. Such a view would be inconceivable to the indigenous people I've studied with. To them, heaven is on Earth, no one is excluded, and death is simply a passage from one state to another, from our "particle" nature to our "wave" nature. Eastern philosophies like Buddhism hold a similar view: consciousness is undying, and paradise is an awakened state here and now.

To the shamans, ultimate healing is not of the physical body only but of the luminous energy field—the light body that takes us beyond this life. This is the body that we will keep with us for a very long time after this life ends, and that we neglect entirely in the West.

Another persistent myth we labor under is a belief in evil as an independent principle in the universe. But far more compelling to me is the view that we live in a benevolent universe that will go out of its way to conspire on our behalf—when we are in right relationship with it and when the hardware in our brain is able to sustain the experience of Oneness.

These old stories linger in what the psychiatrist Carl Jung called the collective unconscious, the repository of ideas and memories shared by our species. The collective mythology runs so deep that we seldom stop to think, *This story has gotten old*. It generally takes global crises, game-changing technologies, and radical discoveries to replace the old myths with new ones. Just as the invention of the printing press altered our worldview in the centuries that followed, the World Wide Web and AI are a transforming narrative of our age. We do not know the new myths that will emerge in the coming decades, but we do know that the old myths have exhausted themselves.

In exploring and finding a new personal mythology, we can invite new forces to touch our lives, preparing us to create a more sustainable future.

Archetypal Energies

At this point in our history, it's pretty clear that the human species needs to be more collaborative, creative, and cooperative—qualities that are aspects of the archetypal Mother figure. To bring balance back into our relationship with Mother Earth and with one another, we need to improve on the masculine mythology of domination, conquest, and hierarchical power. And on a personal level, we need to overcome the self-focused, power-hungry, battle-fixated, dominator mind-set.

It's not enough to simply promise that we'll change our diet and lifestyle and be kinder to ourselves and others. We have to actively engage archetypal energies that will reorient our values and actions. Carl Jung described archetypes as "forms in the psyche which seem to be present always and everywhere."[1] The archetypes we need to draw on are, in fact, very ancient and have guided and influenced human experience throughout time. Archetypes are embedded in mythology handed down through oral tradition, wisdom teachings, and sacred books, and woven into religious and secular rituals. In fact, mythology and folklore based on tales of human interaction with archetypal forces—the gods of old—have existed in every culture since humans first developed language.

I am not asking you to call on the old gods or to go sacrifice some chickens or goats. But I am inviting you to engage the underlying forces of nature that these archetypes represent. When we only expose ourselves to the disempowering myths that have wormed their way into books, movies, and newscasts, we end up reliving them by default. We get caught up in desperately competing with a younger rival; we fall prey to a clever trickster; we repeat habits that make us physically sick, psychologically unwell, and spiritually bereft. Our perception narrows to the tried-and-true, and we lose the ability to creatively interact with life. Stuck in crisis, we fail to recognize an opportunity to view a rival as a partner, or a trickster as a potential playmate. We need to work with the archetypes and their energies differently.

Not too long ago, Mark, a successful stockbroker who believes that there are only so many slices to the pie and you have to grab yours before someone else does, came with me on an expedition to the Andes Mountains. The shamans we were working with pointed out that Mark was accumulating slices of the wrong pie. He was going after the pie that would bring him more money, but the Great Pie, they said, is the pie of wisdom and generosity, and there are plenty of slices to go around.

Their message struck Mark like a slap in the face, and he came to me angry and frustrated, claiming that the Indians only wanted his money, that they were trying to sell him stones and feathers and cloths for their personal gain. He wanted to leave the expedition right away. Fortunately, we were high in the mountains, and there was no way to get down to the valley until the following day. I suggested that what was really upsetting Mark was the realization that no amount of wealth, fame, or notoriety could ever fill his heart and soul. Reluctantly, he agreed that might be true. He acknowledged that his definition of success was killing him, the stress and long hours were taxing his health, and that he had to widen his perspective if he hoped to find any peace of mind, and that this was the reason he had joined our expedition.

Updating your personal mythology means abandoning the seductive yet limiting beliefs that create for each of us a living hell. Mark's belief was that he could help the world only after he became very rich; then he would donate money to charities he liked. It was a shock to realize that if he wanted to find that fulfillment he was seeking, he had to start with changing his personal myth of scarcity, of not having enough to make a difference now. Changing your personal myths requires interacting with familiar stories in new ways so that you can use those energies more wisely. You could revise how you engage with your inner warrior, for example, by giving up judgment toward yourself and others—and reserving your adversarial energy for only the most essential battles and the athletic field.

We can become warriors who fight our own demons instead of looking for people to demonize and dominate. We can wage holy war on the infidel within—or even chuck the warrior energy altogether and see what our inner infidel has to teach us. Similarly, we could work with the pouting inner child who always wants things our way, or the jealous Aphrodite who demands that all attention and adoration be focused on her.

EXERCISE
FINDING AN EMPOWERING MYTHOLOGY

Personal myths are deep and unconscious stories that reveal themselves through dreams and fairy tales. Each of us is the hero or heroine of our own personal mythology, but if your guiding myths are keeping you in bondage to a disempowering worldview, then finding a new personal mythology is essential for you to grow a new body. This is particularly important today when the old myths are bankrupt and the new ones have not yet appeared.

The first step to finding a new narrative is to identify the old myths and stories that no longer serve you. Write a short fairy tale—no more than one page—about a man or woman locked up in a castle dungeon. How did the prisoner come to be there? What are the beliefs and fears keeping him or her there?

Sit quietly and write a new story in which you leave the castle into the unknown, meeting challenges and opportunities, crafting a new destiny. Identify the strengths and beliefs on which your new narrative is based.

Moving Toward a New Mythology

In the next four chapters, we'll look at four myths that illustrate the power that comes with embracing a new personal mythology. The stories of Parsifal, Psyche, Arjuna, and Siddhartha map the steps of the journey to break free of worn-out beliefs and change our destinies. Each of these individuals embarked on a heroic journey of transformation in which they became divine.

Our vehicle for working with these myths and claiming their power is the medicine wheel, a teaching tool from indigenous people of the Americas that is integral to all earth-based spiritual traditions.

Stonehenge in England and Machu Picchu in Peru—ancient sites of the people of Britain and the Andes—are perhaps the most well-known examples of sacred places grounded in the land and the cycles of nature. Dominant features of both sites are massive stones oriented to the yearly movement of the sun as it traverses the sky from spring equinox to summer solstice to autumn equinox to winter solstice, then begins its journey again. Each can be thought of as a great medicine wheel placed on the earth.

The medicine wheel provides a map for tackling the challenges of transformation. As we work our way around the wheel in the four directions—from South to West to North to East—we prepare for growing a new body and crafting a new mythology that will help you get there.

We begin in the South, with the journey of the healer and healing our wounds. We then move to the West and the journey of the Divine Feminine, overcoming our fear of death. From there we move to the North, the journey of the sage, where we learn to be still, like the surface of the lake that reflects everything and disturbs nothing. Finally, we reach the East and the journey of the visionary, where we practice dreaming our world into being.

The journey around the medicine wheel, with the tasks each direction calls us to do, is the classic hero's journey. We are called upon to leave our ordinary existence as we know it and step into the unknown so that we may transform our lives beyond our wildest dreams.

This is a solo journey, in that no one can do the work for you. But that does not mean you walk the medicine wheel alone. You embark on this path as part of a lineage of men and women of wisdom who have come before you. Help from the universe is always available, but you have to humble yourself to benefit from its assistance. Without humility, you will almost certainly slip back into the old ways, into the same disempowering, me-centered stories. The ego wants to take a quick turn around the medicine wheel and be completely renewed, but that is not the way transformation works. You have to master the lessons of each direction.

Chapter 10

THE JOURNEY OF THE HEALER: SHEDDING THE PAST AND HEALING OUR MOTHER WOUNDS

There comes a time in every man's life when he must encounter his past. For those who are dreamed, who have no more than a passing acquaintance with power, this moment is usually played out from their deathbeds as they try to bargain with fate for a few more moments of lifetime.

But for the dreamer, the person of power, this moment takes place alone, before a fire, when he calls upon the specters of his personal past to stand before him like witnesses before the court. This is the work of the healer, where the medicine wheel begins.

— FROM DANCE OF THE FOUR WINDS, BY ALBERTO VILLOLDO AND ERIK JENDRESEN

You may be wondering why I am inviting you to go on a mythic journey to craft a new life. It's because your body and your health are defined as much as by your inner stories and how you love and forgive, as by what you eat. And we all know how difficult it is to change our eating habits. Changing our inner stories is even more challenging. And psychology does not seem to help much. After 100 years of psychotherapy, we have very little to show for it, with a few notable exceptions (like cognitive behavioral therapy). To grow a new body, you also have to grow a new story about your journey through your life as a hero, so that you can stop running on the old programming and worn-out beliefs.

In the southern hemisphere, the Southern Cross constellation occupies a prominent place in the psyche as well as in the sky, much as the Big Dipper and North Star guide residents of the northern hemisphere. The four stars in the Southern Cross orient the stargazer and symbolically reflect the progression through the four stages of the medicine wheel.

The South is considered the domain of the serpent: in indigenous cosmology, the Milky Way is the Sky Serpent. In many cultures the serpent archetype represents sexuality and the life force. Eastern traditions associate the serpent with *kundalini*, a vital force often depicted as a snake coiled at the base of the spine. The serpent represents the instincts and literal thinking: everything is just as we see it, without nuance or ambiguity, summed up in the expression *It is what it is.* In this mode, feeling and emotion are not involved. Like the cold-blooded serpent, we act unsentimentally.

In some situations, seeing through the eyes of the serpent is exactly what's needed. When you're in danger and fear might cause you to panic and make bad choices, acting instinctually can ensure your survival. If you're standing on an open mountaintop with lightning striking around you, it is not a time for reflection but for your serpent instinct to kick in and tell you to find safe ground.

The serpent reminds us of our connection to the earth, the source of our sustenance and support. The physical realm of flesh, soil, and rocks awakens our senses as, like the snake, we outgrow our old skins and leave them behind. The next step is to shed the roles and identities that no longer serve you and trust that you can survive without them. Staying in touch with what your body is sensing, you can act instinctively without deliberating about what to do. A pregnant woman in labor doesn't ruminate on whether or not to give birth; she trusts in her body's innate wisdom and surrenders to the contractions.

Serpent compels us to move forward when we need to shed old identities and make a radical change. If we get stuck in serpent awareness, however, we live mindlessly, concerned with our own well-being and survival without regard for the feelings or needs of others. We cling to what we know—the identities and roles that served us in the past. Very often, these are identities shaped more by our conditioning and the influence of our parents than by any conscious choice on our part. Because the primitive reptilian brain finds comfort in familiarity, under its influence we avoid change, even when the old roles no longer suit us. A person gets married yet isn't fully committed to leaving the old freewheeling, multiple-sexual-partner lifestyle behind. Someone recovers from a life-threatening illness yet remains a medical patient, vulnerable and afraid.

Just as the eyesight of a snake becomes less acute when it's about to shed its skin, our perception tends to narrow as we resist needed change. Seeing danger, not opportunity, we miss the chance to experiment with new ways of being that might make us happier or lead to greater self-discovery.

Robin, a woman in her late 30s who was the mother of two teenage boys, came to me at a crisis point in her life. She was distraught because her teenage sons now seemed to need her only to do their laundry and clean their rooms. Yet she had no identity other than "Mom," and as upset as she was that her role had devolved into being her children's maid, she was even more terrified of what her life would be like if she tried something else—perhaps a job in advertising, her previous career. Robin knew how to design magazine ads for women's clothing, but the field had gone on without her, and she knew nothing about

Internet marketing, search engine optimization, or virtual storefronts.

When she came to my office, Robin complained that life at home was making her angry and sick: she had gained 30 pounds, was prediabetic, and whenever she tried to discipline her sons, her heart started racing and she felt a headache coming on. Every morning she woke up in a daze, unable to think clearly without several cups of coffee. She knew she had to change. I asked her to begin her new diet with the brain foods that repair the hippocampus, explaining that this would help her break free of the old thinking that kept her locked in her role as mother and maid long past the point it was helpful to her children or to her. I also asked her to stay away from gluten and dairy for a month, to see if she was sensitive to either one, and to avoid sugar and refined carbs.

In our next session three weeks later, I lit a large candle that I keep on my desk. I asked Robin to write her most uncomfortable roles on small pieces of paper, then to take each piece, roll it up, blow a prayer into it, and then hold the "stick" in the flame as it burned. Just as her fingertips were beginning to feel the heat from the flame, she was to drop the burning paper into a metal bowl I had filled with sand. I explained that this was an ancient ritual for releasing the worn-out roles that were informing her old identity by symbolically turning them to ashes.

The first role she wanted to release was *maid*. "I am so done with that one!" she practically shouted. Then she burned the roles of *short-order cook, laundrywoman, wife,* and finally *advertising manager.* In shedding that role from her earlier career, she opened herself up to a new role that incorporated both the changes in her industry and the changes in herself. She hoped to use her skills in a new way—perhaps in advertising, perhaps in another field.

Shamans have long known what neuroscientists are now confirming—the power of ritual to change the brain. Small rituals like the one Robin performed help lift your awareness out of your literal, limbic brain into your higher-order neural networks. As Robin committed her old roles to the fire, she let out a big sigh of relief. However, she decided to keep one role—*mother.* "I will be their mom all my life, but no longer the maid," she explained. Had Robin burned her old roles without first repairing her hippocampus, this exercise would have been little more than a quaint gesture based on good intentions. Good intentions are easily forgotten, and willpower can dwindle away, making it extremely difficult to truly shift your mind-set or behavior.

After our session, Robin went home and informed all the men in her family, including her husband, that she was going back to school to learn about Internet marketing. If they wanted to eat, they would have to cook for themselves. If they wanted clean laundry, they would have to learn how to operate the washer and dryer. And Robin stuck with her decision. For two weeks, her house was a disaster area, with dirty dishes and dirty clothes everywhere. But then hunger and hygiene made the men in her household rise to the occasion.

At our next meeting Robin informed me that her blood sugar had stabilized and returned to normal, that she had lost 15 pounds, and that she was loving being back in school.

In the journey of the healer, you have to trust that just as the serpent is protected by nature as it sheds its skin, your soft, vulnerable underbelly will be safe without the roles and identities you discard. As the oldest student in her class at the local community college, Robin found her new direction frightening. And she had to restrain herself from rescuing her husband and boys from their mess. But repairing her hippocampus—the brain center associated with new learning—allowed her to acquire new skills that would help her thrive as a marketing executive rather than simply survive as a housekeeper.

Parsifal and Healing the Masculine

The legend of Parsifal, a knight of King Arthur's Round Table, illustrates a man's archetypal quest for wholeness and healing, the struggle to let go of the identities of the past in order to evolve. For Parsifal, the work of the serpent was to heal the wounded masculine: to embody a new, more enlightened masculinity by integrating his inner feminine—qualities like beauty, feeling, and love that in most men lie dormant and must be actively awakened by their mothers, lovers, or spouses.

Central to the Parsifal legend is the Holy Grail. The embodiment of the sacred feminine, the Grail is the object of Parsifal's quest.

According to the legend, Parsifal—whose name means *innocent fool*—was an infant when his father died. He was raised by his mother in the forests of Wales, sheltered from men and their warrior ways. But in adolescence, he saw a group of knights riding through the woods. With their shining armor and flying banners, they were irresistible to the lad. The urge to become a man and prove his mettle stirred within him, and Parsifal decided to follow the knights on the quest for the Grail.

Parsifal's mother was distraught at the prospect of losing her son. She wanted him to remain forever her boy, safe by her side at home. She knew well that if he became a knight, he would lead a life of conflict, battling enemies in distant lands. "If you must go," she told him, "promise that you will remain chaste and will ask no questions, and that you will always wear this homespun shirt to remind you of your mother and her steadfast love." Being a dutiful son, Parsifal agreed to those conditions. When we're young, we follow the directives of our parents and the dictates of our culture, unaware of how constricting those prescribed roles might come to be in time.

Parsifal set off to find the knights, and as he was leaving the forest, he came upon the maiden Blanchefleur, or "white flower," who was preparing a wedding feast. (Blanchefleur represents the pure feminine energy that exists within everyone, male or female; Parsifal must claim his inner feminine if he is to become a whole man.) But with his mother's words ringing in his ears, Parsifal upheld his vow of chastity and refused to kiss Blanchefleur, instead choosing the life of the warrior. Even today, our young men are initiated by war, not love.

No one at the court took Parsifal seriously when he asked how he, too, could become a knight. King Arthur smiled. "If you can defeat the Red Knight," he told Parsifal, "his horse and armor are yours." To everyone's astonishment, Parsifal not only challenged the Red Knight but won the duel, killing him entirely by accident. This awakened the virile warrior in Parsifal, but behind the swagger, his masculinity was not yet fully formed. Under his armor, he still wore his mother's homespun shirt.

Setting out again, Parsifal came to a castle where the Holy Grail was guarded under the protection of the Fisher King. Wounded in his groin—some versions say because he misused his sexual powers—the Fisher King represents the man whose masculinity is wounded. Because the king was unable to procreate, his land was barren and his subjects were discontent. This is the condition of the modern male who has not been touched by the Grail, and initiated by love. He may work hard to make his family happy, yet he is powerless to do so and feels unappreciated and unloved.

The Fisher King gave Parsifal the Grail Sword. (The sword represents the masculine principle, charged with guarding the Holy Grail, the feminine force.) Then, the king hosted a feast, and at the end of the meal the Grail was brought out. Everyone watched anxiously, for the legend said it would take an innocent young man to ask the question—"Whom does the Grail serve?"—that would release the Grail's power, the elixir that heals all wounds. Alas, when the cup was passed to Parsifal, he didn't recognize it as the Grail. Heeding his mother's plea not to ask questions, he simply passed the cup along. To his uninitiated mind, the vessel was just another cup of wine.

Parsifal woke the next day to find the castle empty and his horse saddled outside. As he rode across the drawbridge, the Grail palace disappeared into the mist behind him. Parsifal went on to rescue damsels in distress and liberate castles under siege, proving his worth as a knight performing the usual heroic deeds. At King Arthur's castle, the Knights of the Round Table welcomed him. But as they were celebrating Parsifal's triumphs, a crone interrupted the revelry. The old woman scolded Parsifal for failing to ask the Grail question, thereby losing the opportunity to release its healing power for the benefit of all mankind. Chastened publicly and ridiculed by the hideous maiden, Parsifal set off to find the Grail castle again and rectify his error. But he wandered for years without success, like many men who cannot find a deep purpose or an abiding love, or a sense of fulfillment.

Finally, in old age, Parsifal met a group of travelers who berated him for wearing his armor on Good Friday, a holy day. The knight removed his armor, and with that he immediately received directions to the Grail castle. There, at last—or so we hope, because the story ends before the conclusion—Parsifal posed the magic question, breaking the spell that had kept his masculinity wounded like the Fisher King's. Drinking from the vessel of pure, healing, feminine power, Parsifal became whole. It is only when a man sheds his armor, his warrior persona, that he can drink from the Grail cup and be healed by the Divine Feminine.

The Holy Grail is what all of us are searching for, men and women alike. The elixir it contains can soothe the wounds inflicted upon us by our violent history and the dictates of our parents and our culture. Like Parsifal, many of us don armor—a business suit or a tough attitude, for example—and head off to battle each morning, freeing castles under siege but receiving no gratitude or satisfaction for our efforts.

As long as Parsifal remained tethered to the past and his identity as a warrior, he couldn't evolve into the man he was meant to be. He couldn't fulfill his promise to retrieve the Grail, so the people of the land suffered. Male or female, when we finally let go of who we think we're supposed to be and shed our fear of disapproval, we open our eyes to new opportunities. We're no longer afraid to be curious, to ask questions, to take risks. But first we have to take off our armor and shed the home-spun mother-garment underneath.

It's daunting to walk away from familiar issues and battles—to put down the sword and remove the emotional armor—but it's a crucial step in our transformation. Without taking this step, we will not recognize the Grail and release its healing power.

We may not even realize that we're holding on to the role of the misunderstood, underappreciated warrior, and continuing to blame our parents for opportunities we didn't have and what we failed to become. But to break out of this victim identity, we have to recognize that our parents, too, lived out the Parsifal myth, as did their parents and the generations before them. The journey of the healer involves breaking the chains of blame and stepping into a new role, writing a new story to free not only ourselves but also future generations.

Throughout our lives, we will continue to shed identities when, like the serpent's skin, they become too tight. Eventually we will discover that all roles are simply suits we hang in the closet, to put on and take off as circumstances require.

Once you've started the work of the South and begun searching for your personal Grail, you're free to be the dreamer instead of the dreamed, the healer instead of the healed, the creator instead of the passive recipient of your life. Next, you will find yourself facing in a new direction on the medicine wheel: West, the way of the jaguar.

EXERCISE
BURNING OLD ROLES AND IDENTITIES

The micro-fire ritual is an effective practice for rewiring the brain and shedding outworn roles and identities, so you can release the constraints of the past and move on. It requires focusing your intent on the task. It is your intent that gives the ritual depth, significance, and transformative power. Remember that the ancient limbic brain changes through the power of ritual.

Traditionally, this ritual involves a group of people gathered around a large fire outdoors, but it can be just as meaningful as a solo rite indoors.

You will need a fat candle at least four inches tall, a box of wooden toothpicks, matches, and a fireproof bowl. (You can fill the bowl partway with sand, if you like.)

Light the candle, and then pick up a toothpick. As you hold it, think of a role or identity that is no longer serving you. Blow gently on the toothpick, envisioning that you are transferring all the feelings of that outmoded role or identity into that small piece of wood. Then hold the toothpick to the candle flame. When you can no longer comfortably hang on to the flaming stick, drop it into the bowl. Continue blowing roles and identities into the toothpicks, one by one, until you have burned up all the stale old roles and identities you need to release.

The first time I did this exercise, I began with the role of *father*. As I brought the stick to the fire, I thanked my father for the love and lessons I had received from him, no matter how flawed they were. I know now that he did his best. I continued the ritual by releasing the role of *son*, and with a prayer, thanked my children for teaching me how to be a son and father. Then I moved on to shedding the identities of *husband, lover, healer, victim*, and so on, until I had burned up nearly 200 roles and identities!

Chapter 11

THE JOURNEY TO THE DIVINE FEMININE: FACING THE FEAR OF DEATH AND MEETING THE GODDESS

Now on a certain day, while Mary stood near the fountain to fill her pitcher, the angel of the Lord appeared unto her, saying, "Blessed art thou, Mary, for in thy womb thou hast prepared a habitation for the Lord. Behold, light from heaven shall come and dwell in thee, and through thee shall shine in all the world."

— THE GOSPEL OF MATTHEW

The Divine Mother, the symbol of the feminine, is found in all cultures, manifesting as the Madonna or Kali or Quan Yin—even as wisdom itself, the mother of all Buddhas. We intend to meet the Divine Feminine in her own domain—the rich, dark, inner world that we journey to when we face our death. This journey is associated with the West direction on the medicine wheel, the place of the jaguar and the dying sun.

When we meet the Divine Feminine in the ordinary world, we are smitten. A man sees the goddess in the woman he falls in love with—until she begins to make his life impossible. When women meet the Divine Feminine in the world, they often idolize or envy her, instead of recognizing her beauty and power within themselves.

The Greek tale of the prince Actaeon and Diana, goddess of the hunt and the moon, illustrates what can happen when we unexpectedly stumble across the Divine Feminine. During a hunt with his hounds and his male friends, Actaeon left his companions resting and wandered off to explore a part of the forest he had never seen. He came upon a valley, thick with pines and cypress, and a pristine stream that flowed into a shallow pool. There, to his surprise and delight, was the beautiful Diana, wading naked as her nymphs bathed her. The goddess had left her bow and quiver of arrows on the riverbank beside her sandals and robe. When the nymphs saw Actaeon they quickly rushed to cover Diana with their own naked bodies, trying to hide the divine form from the young mortal's lustful gaze. But the goddess towered above her nymphs, and she stood proud, revealing her full body to the hunter. Splashing water in his face, she told him, "Now you can say you have seen Diana naked."

With that, antlers suddenly sprang from Actaeon's head; his muscular neck grew longer and sprouted fur; his arms turned into legs and his hands into hooves. Stunned, he bounded away, astonished at how quickly he could run. But when he stopped breathless by a pool and stooped to drink he caught his reflection in the water and saw that he had become a stag. At that instant he heard his own dogs baying and barking, hot on his trail. Terrified, he fled, but the dogs were soon at his heels, the first of them tearing at his flank. Actaeon tried calling their names, but only a strange, guttural sound came out of his mouth. In an instant the dogs felled him, ripping open his underbelly and tearing out his entrails, as he bled to death.

In turning the lustful Actaeon into a stag, the symbol of male virility and power, the goddess transforms him into man's wildest fantasy—the all-fertile stud, the human horned god. In ancient Paleolithic art, medicine men were portrayed as horned beings, like "The Sorcerer" in the famed cave painting at Trois-Frères in Ariège, France. Even today, we refer to all-male gatherings as stag parties. Meanwhile, the goddess is portrayed as granting all wishes—even our deepest, most unconscious ones, which, if we're not careful, may also contain the elements of our demise.

Meeting the Jaguar

The sun sets in the West, bringing forth the cacophony of night in the jungle. In the darkness, a sleek black cat moves silently. The jaguar is a potent symbol of the Divine Feminine. With no predators in the rain forest, the jaguar lives free of fear, taking just what it needs from the jungle for nourishment and no more. It doesn't kill out of greed, or for sport, or out of concern that the food supply will dry up. It doesn't scramble to be more, do more, or accomplish more. It doesn't need to prove itself. The jaguar hunts, explores, and sleeps as required, living a secure and balanced life.

To indigenous peoples in the southwestern United States, the Mexican jungles, and the Andean highlands, the jaguar symbolizes the transforming power of One Spirit Medicine in much the same way that the caduceus—the staff with two intertwined serpents crowned by eagle wings—symbolizes healing to Western physicians. In fact, the earliest civilization in the Americas, that of the Olmec of Mexico, was so fascinated with the jaguar that this great feline is depicted in much of Olmec art, including many figures that are half-human, half-jaguar.

For the Maya, the jaguar is a symbol of death and acceptance of death's role in the cycle of life. Before the Spanish conquest, the Maya high priests were called balams—*balam* is Maya for jaguar—indicating they had traveled through the domains beyond death. They had made the symbolic journey to the underworld, conquered their fear of death, and returned with the elixir of immortality. In our journey to the Divine Feminine, we embody the wisdom of the jaguar, letting go of our fear of the unknown and trusting that what is dying inside us is what needs to be renewed in order to serve all life. With the cycle of life and death, harmony is reestablished. All species flourish as part of the balance of nature.

For us, the promise of the jaguar is to feel at home and safe regardless of any danger that surrounds us. The jaguar helps you discover fearlessness, and that life provides you with everything you need to maintain your health and inner peace. Jaguar gives you the confidence to step out and boldly explore the unknown and not cling to the familiar, sure that you're headed where you need to go and that you're moving in synch with your life's purpose. Jaguar medicine brings you into balance and sanity—even if the world around you seems to have gone mad. Jaguar medicine returns your power and confidence and restores your health.

If you allow jaguar to guide you far enough, she will lead you to the realm of the goddess to receive her wisdom directly. You may have experienced this as you recovered from an illness or accident—the deep sense of gratitude at being healthy or able to walk once again. And if you have ever known someone to say, "My cancer saved my life," you know what I mean. This person not only recovered their health but also found a new life direction infused with meaning and wisdom.

If you complete this step on the medicine wheel, meeting the goddess and facing the fear of death, you can become like the jaguar, living with creativity and grace and experiencing wellness and balance. You can even hope to defeat death, like the ancient Mayan wisdom keepers, by discovering your eternal nature.

To understand this concept of defeating death, we need to consider the philosophy of the ancient Americans. They believed, as many people still do, that we have an essence that continues beyond death. But contrary to our religious thinking, in which the eternal nature of the soul is assumed, the shamans of old held that immortality is merely a seed, a potential that we all possess but one we have to awaken and empower to ensure the continuity of our consciousness beyond death. Our life, therefore, must be dedicated to spiritual practice—so that we can learn how to "leave this life alive," as the Amazon shamans say. The Maya called this process *the awakening of your jaguar body,* and the balams, the priests who had mastered it, were the cartographers of the afterlife, and drew the maps to the realms beyond death with the same accuracy and precision that we draw maps of our physical landscape. The Tibetan Buddhist equivalent of the jaguar body is the *light body.* One effect of completing the journey through the medicine wheel is to germinate the seeds of immortality you carry inside you.

You might ask, *What does this have to do with growing a new body?*

Everything. Because the jaguar medicine of the ancients is the antidote to fear, and fear, particularly the fear of death, is at the root of every malady. To heal ourselves, and to maintain our health, we must become fearless.

Discovering Your Mortality

Do you remember the first time you thought about your own death? The first time you realized the fact that you will die? In adolescence we feel impervious to death, believing it's something that happens to others but will never happen to us. And so, after one too many beers we drive down winding mountain roads with a carful of friends, denying that the laws of physics apply to us as we careen around the curves without giving safety a second thought. And then one day we lose a loved one or have an accident or a health scare, and we realize that death has always been by our side.

Actually, we have *two* great awakenings to our mortality. The first is the one that occurs when we grasp that we're temporal beings and that one day, our time on Earth will end. If we take this awareness to heart, from that moment on we know that every moment is precious. Then, our lives are forever changed.

The second great awakening happens when we *master* our fear of death. This arrives with the understanding that our nature is trans-temporal—outside of time—and undying, continuing for all eternity. Our understanding of our infinite nature cannot be merely an intellectual one. It must be a visceral awareness, a knowing at a cellular level. In many preagricultural societies, there is a rite of initiation to foster this awareness, a symbolic encounter with death in which the initiate experiences the seamless continuity of life beyond physical existence.

Whether or not you consciously experience a symbolic death in a rite of initiation, or a close call after an accident or health crisis, mastering the fear of death is immensely liberating, freeing you to use your creative faculties to find harmony in the chaos of everyday existence. The cacophony of the jungle becomes music. A tragedy becomes the foundation of a new and more fulfilling way of living. You start to envision a more enriching life for yourself and a more sustainable future for your community. You are called to serve the earth and all living beings, as you realize that we will continue together for eons to come.

After you've started the work of the jaguar, the new stories you write for yourself will be invigorating, extending beyond mere concern for your immediate survival needs. But be warned: If you try to rush the process by pushing aside your fear of death without confronting it, or scrambling to figure your way out of a health crisis as quickly as possible by finding every medical expert in the field, the initiation will be incomplete. The close brush with death will seem like a lucky break, not an invitation to discover your undying nature. The problems you thought you had left behind will in all likelihood return, as you return to fear-based behaviors of the past. When the challenge of the jaguar remains unmet, life again becomes overwhelming, with no time left for the really important things.

To master fear, we need to return it to its rightful role as nature's early warning system, not as a habitual state of being. Fear alerts us to possible danger in our surroundings, making us ready to respond appropriately. But when fear settles into the nervous system instead of passing through it, we become possessed by it. The HPA axis goes into hyperdrive. Life turns chaotic at every level. The death clock inside every cell cannot keep accurate time any longer. Stress hormones flood our brain and we cannot grow a new body because we cannot access the higher order neural networks in the brain.

From the standpoint of biology, health is determined by the degree of harmony and complexity in the body. Nature favors complexity. The human being evolved from a single-celled organism into a highly specialized creature. But complexity alone is not enough to create health: the system must be coherent and harmonious as well. A hundred people playing a hundred different musical instruments do not make an orchestra. To create music these instruments have to play in harmony.

The more complex and coherent the systems in your body, the healthier you will be. An example is heart rate variability—naturally occurring fluctuations in the rhythm of the heartbeat—which is one measure of overall health. The more variable your heart rate, the healthier your heart, and the more harmoniously all the systems in your body work together, the greater your resilience and health.

This understanding of coherence and complexity is reflected even in health at the cellular level. Orderly cells create health while disorderly cells revert back to a primitive state and begin to form tumors. Chaotic cells steal nourishment from the body and unlike healthy cells, refuse to die. They defy the instructions from the mitochondria—that control the cells' "death clock"—to die so that younger, more vital cells can replace them. When cells lose their complexity, they can no longer feed on healthy fats but only on sugars—which is why eliminating all sugars and carbohydrates from your diet is so important for healing from cancer and other disease.[1]

As cancerous cells multiply in the body, they wreak havoc, ultimately killing the host that is feeding them. And what happens at a cellular level is reflected in what happens to your life if you refuse to accept endings as a natural part of life. When fear of death takes over, it determines what your experiences will be, eventually sucking the life out of you.

Endings, Transitions, and Beginnings

We have to let ourselves be terrified by the transition that the death of the old ushers in. Fear of death (whether death of the body, a way of thinking, a relationship, a situation, or a dream) has to be faced fully and consciously—and then overcome—for new, healthy growth to take place.

At just 12 years old, Annie was the youngest cancer patient I had ever worked with. Her parents had brought her to see me in the hope that we could heal her brain cancer. They had tried every conceivable medical intervention to no avail and were looking to me for the cure they had failed to find anywhere else. Annie had lost all her hair from chemotherapy and looked like a young, smiling Buddha as she sat in a big leather chair in my office.

I explained to Annie's parents the difference between healing and curing. While curing is the elimination of symptoms, healing works at a much deeper level, treating the causes of the imbalance that lead to disease. And while a cure is the ideal outcome of a medical intervention, healing is the product of a journey in which all aspects of your life are transformed—even if you end up dying. You carry your healed self into your next life.

I asked Annie's parents to sit outside in the waiting area so I could be alone with her. After a few moments of small talk, she told me bluntly, "I'm not afraid." She went on to say that angels came to her every night in her dreams—and even, sometimes, during the day. But her parents were afraid for her. "I can't tell them about the angels," Annie said. But she thought I would understand. And I did. I sensed that the veils between the worlds were parting for Annie and that she was preparing for the great journey home. But her parents were understandably determined to do everything possible to help Annie live, and this meant trying to get rid of her cancer by taking her to a string of specialists and finally, as a last resort, to me.

I've been around long enough to understand that death is part of life. And some of my most successful healings consisted of helping my clients die peacefully and consciously. So I performed an Illumination on Annie to help bring balance to her energy field and thus to her body. The Illumination is the core healing practice of shamanic energy medicine. In an Illumination, the luminous energy field is cleared of the imprints of disease to help mobilize the body's own healing systems.

Annie's doctors had not given her long to live. But I know that death is a doorway to continued life in the world of Spirit. I worked on clearing the stale energies that had accumulated in her field, helping to lighten her load for the great journey ahead of her. As she lay on my treatment table, she went into a deep sleep.

At the end of our session, Annie returned to the leather chair that almost seemed to swallow her, a smile on her face. "Am I going to be okay?" she asked me, and we both knew what she was talking about. "Yes," I said. "You're going to be just fine." And then she asked me how she could help her mother and father. "They're really afraid," she said. I'm always stunned by the wisdom of many children—and equally stunned by the lack of wisdom in so many adults.

When Annie's parents came back into the room, they found both of us smiling. I told them what great work their daughter had done. I suggested they eliminate all gluten from Annie's diet, as well as sugar, dairy, and all possible allergens. Then I recommended that she take omega-3 fatty acids daily to help rebuild the regions in the brain that had been damaged by chemo. We know how to die in the same way that we know how to be born, and it helps to have our neural apparatus in the best working order possible.

I learned that Annie passed away a few months later with a smile on her face, in the arms of her angels.

Love and Letting Go

The forest undergrowth and the canopy above can't thrive unless the soil is replenished by the dying plants. Even the jaguar will die, nourishing the tree that will feed the monkey that the next jaguar will feast on. The balance of life in the forest wouldn't be possible without death, just as we can't live in a state of harmony with our environment unless endings are a part of our lives. Things have to die for new things to be born. Death and life are always inexplicably intertwined.

The lesson of the jaguar is to find a balance between, on the one hand, engaging life aggressively and seizing opportunity at all costs and, on the other, approaching life with acceptance and receptivity so we can surrender to the larger creative process. It's a delicate dance between active masculine and receptive feminine. The jaguar teaches us that we can stop hoarding, stop taking more than we need, because Mother Earth will provide us with plenty. We can trust that what lies ahead around a blind corner may actually be better than what we see now.

The medicine of the jaguar allows us to start living more optimistically and imaginatively. Then, instead of worrying about the sun setting, we can enjoy the evening stars and look forward to the sun rising again at just the right time. The obsession with losing what we have—our youth, our belongings, our loved ones, our health—begins to fade. Our relationship with death becomes a healthy one.

Entropy is the law of physics that says that everything in the universe is moving toward chaos and disorder, toward death. Temporary disorder and disorientation are necessary preludes to reorganization at a higher level. This is what we experience when we begin a new relationship, a new career, or a new health plan. Change holds danger but also the potential for something new—and better—to be born.

In the West direction on the medicine wheel, we come to terms with the cycle of destruction and rebirth, the natural order of the universe. We grasp at a deep level that creative chaos can lead to greater harmony and balance. In Hinduism, the cycle of destruction and rebirth is represented in the three principal deities controlling the cosmos: Brahma the creator, Vishnu the preserver, and Shiva the destroyer.

Once we face our fear and experience the sense of loss and despair in every bone in our body, no longer denying it or running away from it, the fear dissipates. Then we can immerse ourselves in the chaos of creation, the primordial soup from which new life arises. There is no dipping a toe into the pool cautiously: total immersion is the only way to experience full initiation into a new stage of being and perceiving. Allowing ourselves to be truly terrified by the unknown, we can let go of the safety of the shore and plunge into unfamiliar waters, aware of the risks but excited by the possibilities.

When we discover that death is part of life, we are able to love more freely. Many of us hesitate to surrender fully to loving another because we fear losing the loved one. In my late 20s, after suffering what I called chronic heartbreak, I vowed never again to be involved in a committed love relationship. The pain of losing the person I was so deeply attached to was too great to bear. And then, after a couple of emotionally barren years, I realized how futile my vow was. One day, after reading a poem of Rumi's, I decided to face my fear. Rumi said to his beloved, "For I have ceased to exist, only you are here." This was the complete opposite of what I had sought in all my earlier relationships: my mantra then was, "For you have ceased to exist, only I am here." Gradually I began to understand, as Rumi did, that in reality all love is, at bottom, a longing for Spirit, for the true Beloved.

Lessons from Myths of the Underworld

Overcoming the fear that holds us back from a new dream is a universal theme in all great stories.

In Greek mythology, the underworld was a place filled with malevolent spirits, rivers with magical powers, and a queen who ruled the shadowy realm and knew its secrets. The underworld also held deeply buried riches and profound wisdom, different from the treasures to be found on the surface. Among the mortals who, according to legend, entered the underworld while alive and emerged unscathed was Hercules, who had the strength to overpower the three-headed guard dog Cerberus.

Courage and strength allowed Hercules to survive what seemed like a fatal mission. In the Greek underworld you attained eternal happiness if you had earned it in the course of your life. The beast Cerberus made sure that you could never return from the realm of Hades once you entered. Hercules's defeating of the guardian dog symbolically opened the passage for other courageous mortals to journey to the unknown to find the truly deep treasures. It required courage for Hercules to meet his fear and breathe into the emotion rather than run away from it. And we are challenged to do the same.

To receive the healing gifts of the Divine Feminine, we can look to another mortal, Psyche, who descended to the underworld and survived. Psyche is the Greek word for *soul,* and her story describes the journey that everyone, male or female, must take if they seek to defeat death and be initiated by love.

The youngest and loveliest daughter of a king, Psyche was so beloved by everyone that Aphrodite, the old goddess of love, became jealous and drove all of Psyche's suitors away. The king consulted an oracle, who told him that he must chain his daughter to a rock to be courted by and married to Death, a horrible monster. The myth tells us that the young, innocent part of ourselves—full of fresh ideas and the opportunities they bring—threatens the old ways. Psyche's challenge was to face Death, and she did, but not in the way she thought she would.

Aphrodite sent her son Eros (Cupid) to shoot an arrow of love into Psyche so that the maiden would be irresistibly attracted to Death. But just as Eros was about to carry out his mother's wishes, he became so distracted by Psyche's beauty that he pricked himself with one of his arrows and fell in love with her himself. He swept Psyche away to his palace in the mountains, defying the threats of his mother, who believed that Psyche's beauty and vitality must be destroyed. As the myth points out, this is precisely what fear of death and loss can do—destroy our beauty and vitality.

Eros was kind and loving to Psyche with one caveat: she was never to look at him. Not wanting to reveal he was a god, he came to her only after dark. Psyche agreed to the conditions and delighted in her unseen husband. But when her sisters came to visit, envious of Psyche's good fortune, they persuaded her to disobey her husband's orders. "What if he's a monster?" they asked.

Psyche hadn't been afraid of the unknown before, but after her sisters' warning, fear got the better of her. She went to bed with a plan. After making love to her husband and letting him fall asleep, she quickly lit a lamp so she could see his face and form. She discovered the beautiful Eros sleeping sweetly and was overjoyed to see he wasn't a monster after all. But then, a drop of hot oil from the lamp fell on Eros's shoulder, and he woke up. Furious that Psyche had disobeyed him, he flew away. In giving in to her own fear amid social pressure from her sisters, she destroyed her happy life.

Psyche entreated the gods for help, but they all feared Aphrodite. In fact, gods are no help in a situation like this, for they are bound to tradition and the old ways. The gods told the devastated Psyche that the only way she could right the situation was to get into Aphrodite's good graces. Though terrified, Psyche took their advice and bravely approached her mother-in-law. She was ready for the work of the West: confronting and overcoming her fears.

Aphrodite, however, was furious that Psyche had dared to approach her. She then assigned Psyche four impossible tasks she had to complete if she wanted her husband back. The first was to sort a huge pile of seeds before nightfall; if Psyche failed, she would die. This task represents our fear of time running out. *How will we have time to accomplish everything in our lives? How can we sort what's important from what isn't? Will we have enough time for the things that really matter to us? What if time runs out?*

With the help of a colony of ants who persevered through the night, Psyche managed to complete the task. The ants represent the assistance that is always available to us if we look. None of us can do the seemingly impossible alone.

Psyche's second task was to cross a river and retrieve the fleece from the fierce magical rams grazing in a field. The rams represent our fear of adversaries and situations more powerful than we are. We all have to face these adversaries in the form of bosses and family and other obligations in life. Once again, Psyche completed the task with help. The reeds growing on the riverbank told her to wait until dusk when the rams fell asleep; then, she could collect the fleece that had stuck to the reeds when the rams rubbed against them, without risking discovery by the sheep. By allowing the situation to resolve itself, Psyche freed herself from the need to take on an adversary who would easily overpower her.

The third task was to fill a crystal goblet with water from the source of the River Styx, a sacred spring high on a mountain that was protected by sleepless dragons. This was an impossible task for a mortal. Even the gods would be leery of such an assignment. In the course of our lives, we all face seemingly impossible tasks. And when we fear we're not smart enough, good enough, strong enough, or brave enough to handle them, we're like Psyche facing the unattainable. She despaired until an eagle appeared, took the goblet in its talons, flew to the mountaintop, filled the goblet with water from the sacred spring and brought it back to her, helping her accomplish the superhuman task. The eagle, soaring high in the sky, represents the overarching vision, the attention to the big picture, that is necessary to overcome our fears, coupled with the daring to go where ordinary birds would never fly. In the same way, as we upgrade our brain and begin to perceive wholes instead of fragmented parts, we overcome our fear and aim high, taking on greater tasks and challenges than we feel we are capable of. Like the ants and reeds, the eagle represents the helpful forces the universe provides, the synchronous events that occur in our lives when we have the courage to take risks despite our fear.

Psyche's fourth task was to descend into the underworld and ask Persephone for some of her precious beauty cream to give Aphrodite. Frightened beyond words, Psyche decided to take her own life, a guaranteed one-way ticket to the realm of the dead. She climbed an abandoned stone tower and was just about to jump when the tower told her where to find the entrance to the underworld, advising her to carry two coins and two barley cakes with her, and to neither accept assistance from any shades she met in the underworld nor give assistance to anyone who asked her for it. This is the most valuable advice anyone can give us on a journey to conquer fear. We must bring gifts—our abilities and strengths, and qualities like generosity and compassion—and we must be careful who we ask to help us. Even friends who have our best interests at heart often can't or won't provide the assistance or advice we need. Although tempted to help the shades who cried out to her, Psyche followed orders and ignored their pleas. She paid Charon the ferryman, fed the guard dog Cerberus, and accepted only a snack, not a banquet, from Persephone. At last, she successfully retrieved the jar of beauty cream for Aphrodite. Despite her natural urge to help others, Psyche stayed on task, just as we have to focus on our own initiation and not allow ourselves to be diverted by other people's needs as a way of avoiding the inner work we must do.

Psyche was on the verge of successfully completing her tasks, when she gave in to temptation. She peeked inside the jar she was carrying and instantly fell asleep. In her impatience, she tried to rush the process of her initiation, and as a result, slipped back into sleep. Psyche returned to the world with the beauty cream intact, but the gods became jealous and took it away to keep her from sharing the secret of eternal youth with other humans. In the end, Psyche was rescued by Eros—the force of love, which has the power to restore life. Psyche's deep sleep represents the death of her old, limited sense of self that had to be left behind in the land of the dead. When she awakened, she was granted immortality by Zeus.

She had to face her fear of death so she could transform her life. This has always been the central theme of initiation, whether a young man faces this fear in the battlefield, or a woman during childbirth.

All initiation involves a journey to the realm of death and a meeting with the Divine Feminine from which you return renewed. This isn't like the superficial change that comes from making minor tweaks in your life. The journey to the Divine Feminine, like Parsifal's quest for the Grail, is demanding. You have to endure the fear of remaining in the underworld in deep reflection, confronting your own darkness, before you can emerge to light and clarity. If you think what you bring back is just salve for your wounds, you miss the point. The cream isn't ordinary wrinkle cream—or a souvenir on par with a T-shirt or tote bag printed with the slogan *I went to Hades and back!* The beauty cream brings rejuvenation and reinvention. The elixir of immortality is the prize for completing the work of the West.

There is no rushing the journey of initiation. Mastering the fear of death is a lifelong process. You may be challenged and tested many times, although with each time, the way becomes easier.

Once you have reclaimed the ability to renew yourself, you're ready for the next direction on the medicine wheel, the North. There, you will learn to become still so you can retrieve lost aspects of your soul.

Meditate with Jaguar

Jaguars are masters of meditation. Have you ever watched a cat lounging in the sun? Cats know perfect relaxation. A jaguar in the rain forest perches on the lower branches of a tree and watches the world go by, undisturbed by the monkeys and the macaws, completely at ease yet totally alert, with only the tip of its tail twitching now and then. The jaguar teaches us how to relax, deeply relax. (Try explaining to your cat that there are important things to worry about.)

Today we understand that much of the imbalance and disease in our bodies is caused by our inability to slow down and release stress. Our nervous system is designed to provide us with the reflexes to fight or flee when we're in danger. Cortisol and adrenaline flood the bloodstream to give us a burst of energy to deal with threats. But these powerful chemicals are not meant to course through the body for more than a short time. If we're truly in danger, we fight or flee and then quickly recover, as the adrenaline and cortisol are reabsorbed into the body's system and our breathing slows to normal. But when we're chronically on high alert, paralyzed with anxiety, toxic levels of these stress hormones remain in the body, causing inflammation and neuron damage and, ultimately, disease. Instead of mastering our fear of death, our fear of death masters us. Our jaguar climbs to the uppermost branches of the tree like a terrified kitten—and we're powerless to call the fire department to bring it down.

All of us will die someday; however, we don't have to experience the slide to death prematurely. We can master our fear of death so that our lives are not dictated by dread and we are not constantly responding as if a jungle beast were poised to pounce on us at any minute. We can return to a balanced, calm, relaxed state, and be like graceful jaguars, savoring our newly discovered visceral wisdom about the infinite nature of life.

After starting the Grow a New Body program, you will find it much easier to maintain your equilibrium no matter what is happening around you. You won't have a brain full of toxins or a gut overpopulated with Candida sending you back into the old emotional responses. Whatever uncertainties you face, you will find your eyes are now open to opportunities for experiencing something better. You will have the inner resources that serve you in creating a life of your own making.

Chapter 12

THE JOURNEY OF THE SAGE: BECOMING STILL IN MIDAIR

[Behold] many wonders that no one has ever seen before. . . .
Behold the whole universe, the moving and the unmoving, and
whatever else you may desire to see, all within My body. . . .
But with these eyes of yours you cannot see Me. I give you a
divine eye; behold, now, my sovereign yoga-power.

— Bhagavad Gita, Stephen Mitchell translation

When the ancestors of the native peoples of the Americas migrated from Asia, they brought with them a body of wisdom acquired during their long residence in the foothills of the Himalayas. According to molecular archeologists who track variations of mitochondrial DNA, a dozen or so courageous travelers crossed the great Siberian plains to Beringia, a land mass that covered what is now the Bering Strait between Russia and Alaska. They then descended through North and Central

America to the Andes, and from there all the way south to Tierra del Fuego, at the tip of South America. Along the way they built cliff dwellings in the American Southwest and citadels among the clouds like Machu Picchu. In Andean mythology, therefore, the North is the direction of the ancestors. The way of the sage is associated with the North on the medicine wheel and with age-old practices of stillness.

The North is not just the direction of the great sages of the past but also where we experience calm in the midst of furious activity. The North Star is the only still point in a moving sky. The North is associated with the hummingbird, which appears to be perfectly still even as it beats its wings rapidly to remain suspended in midair. Some species of hummingbirds migrate from Canada to South America every fall, flying thousands of miles over the vast ocean. So from the hummingbird we also learn that with stillness comes the ability to go boldly into uncharted territory and make our lives an epic journey regardless of how many oceans we have to cross.

The way of the sage hones our ability to transcend the restless activity of the mind obsessed with the challenges, dramas, and mundane details of everyday life and remain at peace with whatever is happening within and around us. We begin to see order at the heart of uncertainty and tranquility in the eye of the storm. Abandoning fixed ideas about how things should be, we instead take delight in watching plans manifest and dissolve in kaleidoscopic fashion, arranged and rearranged by the vagaries of everyday life. It is in the North that we learn to embrace the Yiddish proverb "Man plans, God laughs."

The sense of inner peace that arises as we start the work of the sage is the direct result of a radical shift in perception. Only when we've stopped grasping and yearning, avoiding and worrying, endeavoring and battling can we find equanimity. In stillness, we can access the wisdom of the ancestors. This is the wisdom that Psyche retrieved from Persephone, knowledge we acquire only in the non-ordinary world, where we experience timelessness in every cell of our being. The gift of the North is stillness in motion.

From the perspective of neuroscience, the sagacity of the North is the wisdom that allowed us to survive without the teeth and claws of stronger, more nimble animals, and later to discover the wonders of science, sending the Hubble Space Telescope into orbit and positing string theory to explain what the universe is made of. We find signs of this newfound wisdom around 50,000 years ago, when our ancestors began to paint the mystical representations of their world on the walls of caves at Lascaux in France and Altamira in Spain. However, if used unwisely, this wisdom can also be employed to make war and wreak havoc—destructive power that was probably unleashed shortly after *Homo sapiens* discovered cave painting, as we eliminated our Neanderthal cousins. The wisdom we find in the North moves us to feel joy, compassion, and empathy—sentiments that lift us beyond the lurid tales of who did what to whom that occupy our more primitive mind.

The gifts of the sage are accessible to us when we stop and see that we've been going a hundred miles an hour yet getting nowhere, and doing a million things yet achieving nothing. Initially, the way of the sage seems like the easiest direction on the medicine wheel to master, given the instructions: *Sit back! Relax! Enjoy the view!* But you can't get to the North without healing your inner masculine—and the drive to achieve power and fame at the expense of others—in the South, and journeying beyond death to meet the Divine Feminine in the West. And when you reach the North, you will most likely find that doing nothing is harder than it looks. And staying still is not an end itself but the necessary ground, the fundamental practice, for witnessing the universe unfolding in our lives in Oneness. In the journey of the sage we acquire that divine eye that allows us to comprehend the entire nature of the Cosmos. But to acquire this kind of vision requires stillness.

With our hectic lives today, being still feels next to impossible. We're so used to multitasking and tracking continual input from our digital devices that quieting the mind for more than a few seconds is a Herculean task. Even when we meditate, focusing on our breathing, we can't resist the urge to scratch an itch, adjust our posture, or curse ourselves for not turning off the text alert on our cell phone.

It is the nature of the mind to jump about, and the overactive mind has been the focus of meditation masters since ancient times. But our minds today are the product of a toxic brain and even more restless, flitting from topic to topic with the dizzying speed of jump cuts in an action film. But with the Grow a New Body program, you can slow the inner movie and quiet the internal racket. And you will be able to access the vast reservoir of wisdom that is humanity's ancestral memory bank.

In the North we learn that what we call reality is an illusion, albeit one we are jointly re-creating in every instant—"What is reality anyway? Nothing but a collective hunch," as the comedian Lily Tomlin put it. *What is* is the product of the map of reality you carry inside you. If you want to change your reality, you need to change the map.

Neuroscientists believe this map is embedded in the neural networks of the brain. Shamans believe it resides in the topography of the luminous energy field. But regardless of where your model of the world resides, to bring about change in your world, and comprehend modern technology and timeless spirituality, you will need to upgrade the quality of your map—exchange the outmoded model for a better one. If, like so many of us in this culture, you are relying on a fear-ridden, scarcity-laden map running on limited bandwidth to navigate through life, the experience of the medicine wheel and the sage teachings will allow you to replace it with a vast and liberating map that includes the entire universe. This is what the warrior Arjuna discovers in his dialogue with the god Krishna, which forms the central narrative of the ancient Hindu text the Bhagavad Gita.

Arjuna: The Challenge to Be Still and Meet God

The Bhagavad Gita was written at a time when the Indian subcontinent was rife with conflict between royal families. As the narrative begins, the archer Arjuna is preparing to do battle against a formidable army of his relatives. It is Arjuna's duty to fight, but he is deeply conflicted at the prospect of battling his own kin. War in this legend is a metaphor for the challenges involved in dealing with the conflicts of human existence, and Krishna, in his advice to Arjuna, imparts timeless wisdom for quieting the inner turmoil we all face. Only when we still the inner war can we receive the wisdom of the universe.

Arjuna cries out to Krishna, who is acting as his charioteer, to help him avoid the battle that will surely result in death and suffering for all. Just as both sides are about to charge, Krishna stops the action, like a director freezing the frame of an epic film just before the bloodshed begins. Like Arjuna, we find it almost impossible to gain any perspective on our lives when we're embroiled in a battle with our boss or spouse or children—even in a fight for our health—and we're trying to sort out what to do. When we become still in the midst of the turmoil, we can observe clearly how our actions and the actions of others, past and present, fit together in the tapestry of life. In the timeless instant when we stop moving and simply witness the moment, the dust settles and the big picture emerges. Then, with this new map of reality in hand, we can choose wisely what course to pursue.

With both armies frozen in mid-motion, Krishna shows Arjuna how the restless mind deceives us. Reflecting on this, Arjuna says:

The mind is restless, unsteady,

turbulent, wild, stubborn;

truly, it seems to me

as hard to master as the wind.[1]

Struggle is a part of life, Krishna tells Arjuna, but we have to resist getting caught up in the dramas we create around our struggles. Then we can take whatever action is necessary "without any thought of results, / open to success or failure."[2]

Our ordinary mental maps can help us figure out how to navigate everyday life, but there are times when their limitations are clear. Whenever our survival programs in the limbic brain are running the show, our emotions and hard-core beliefs get in the way. When that happens, we need to stop and find stillness, to hear a higher voice. Then we realize that Spirit has been with us all along, steering our chariot true, just as Krishna steers Arjuna's.

Krishna tells Arjuna:

For the man who wishes to mature,

the yoga of action is the path;

for the man already mature,

serenity is the path.[3]

Like the hummingbird flying across the ocean in response to a distant calling, we can rely on our inner guidance to lead us safely to the other shore. Krishna explains to Arjuna that everything we do can become an offering to the divine. Sometimes when we're pulled off course, it's because we're meant to experience something other than what we planned. Spirit may have ideas for our life that don't make sense to us at first. There is a greater order that is invisible to humans, Krishna tells Arjuna, and we can align ourselves with this higher plan.

In stillness, we can receive as much guidance from Spirit as we are willing to invite. Sometimes all we want to know is how to respond to our lover or our child; other times we may be ready to learn the deeper nature of reality and the cosmos. We can set the bar at whatever level we want. We may be called to action or to nonaction. (Nonaction doesn't mean doing nothing but rather making a conscious choice not to intervene, allowing situations that can resolve themselves on their own to do so.) Not acting can be even more powerful than acting: it requires great strength not to make a move or react or rescue someone. When we choose to refrain from action and remain still, the fabric of reality is revealed to us and we recognize its awesome precision.

Perceiving the hidden fabric of life is true wisdom. Knowing how we fit into the grand story as co-weavers of this fabric gives us the perspective of the sage.

Since most of us are unlikely to meet a Krishna, how can we witness the vast workings of creation? In the West we're more likely to look to science than to Spirit. The French anthropologist Claude Lévi-Strauss said that for us to know the workings of the universe, we first have to understand the workings of a blade of grass: how photosynthesis transforms light into life and how the roots of that blade of grass absorb minerals from the earth. An indigenous person, however, approaches the matter from a different perspective: for him to know the workings of a blade of grass, he first has to know intuitively the workings of the universe—how suns are created and how galaxies are formed. Today, maybe for the first time in history, we have the opportunity to do both.

One of the most effective ways of quieting manic mental activity and finding stillness is to pay attention to the space between breaths. It's in the pause—the moment between inhaling and exhaling—where you find stillness. Breathing is an autonomic response, and we can't stop it altogether or we die. But we can change the rate of respiration. Breathing practices, many of them ancient techniques, are designed to bring the mind into a state of tranquility and balance. We have the power to cultivate equanimity by consciously controlling the breath.

As you cultivate stillness, everyday challenges will cease to assume crisis proportions. When you're able to take a more sagely view, the world becomes a place of abundance that supports a rich and rewarding life. The frenetic race to get ahead gives way to an awareness that life doesn't have to be a struggle. In the North, you are called to bring beauty and peace to yourself and the world. How best to carry out this mission may not be immediately apparent, but as you continue to practice stillness, it will be revealed to you. All you need to do is make a commitment to be in service, and then let Spirit take care of the details.

Pilgrimage: A Journey of the North

A few years ago, I met a woman, Chloe, who was engaged in a battle for her health. She chose to make a pilgrimage, a practice that was once commonplace, especially in Europe during the Middle Ages. Her pilgrimage was going to take her to northwestern Spain, where she planned to retrace the steps of the apostle Santiago—Saint James—who walked from the Mediterranean to Santiago de Compostela, a journey of some 500 miles.

A pilgrimage involves a geographical destination, and the Camino de Santiago, or Way of Saint James, has been popular for centuries among pilgrims who walk all or part of the route. But a pilgrimage is more than a trek through the countryside; it's also an inner journey, a time of self-reflection. Many travelers dedicate the journey to something larger than themselves. Chloe hoped her pilgrimage would give her a renewed sense of purpose and clarity that would allow her to meet the health challenges she faced.

Soon after she began her journey, Chloe thought she heard a faint voice telling her that she should fast for three days, drinking only water, and then eat for three days, alternating the two for the entire journey. By the time she arrived in Santiago de Compostela three months later, she had recovered her health. While she attributes her recovery to divine intervention, I'm sure that the fasting helped turn on all her body's repair systems. She had intuitively discovered the key to growing a new body, cycling between protein days and no protein (in her case, no food). And the stillness and serenity she discovered allowed her to understand the lessons that her health challenge had brought her.

You don't need to walk the Camino de Santiago to reap the healing benefits of a pilgrimage. You could turn your daily commute to work or a visit to your estranged daughter or, like Chloe, the path back to wellness into a pilgrimage. Whatever the journey, it will have an outer component, with obstacles you have to surmount, and an inner component that involves surrender, discovery, and most likely emotional challenges, as you open yourself to redrawing your maps of reality. Once you have clarity on the greater map for your life and your destiny, you can take the necessary action to align yourself with the new destination.

This pilgrimage is a solo vision quest. The seeker primes his brain with a combination of fasting and superfoods. Then he goes deep into the forest or another natural setting and opens to divine guidance.

The vision quest is the last, all-important step for growing a new body, and you'll find instructions for setting up your own in Chapter 14. But first you must finish the journey around the medicine wheel and follow the path of the visionary in the East.

EXERCISE
I AM MY BREATH

Traditional practices for cultivating stillness and equanimity involve meditating with the breath. This exercise is effective for quieting the restless mind.

Sit in a darkened room with a small candle lit before you. As you gaze at the candle, note that your awareness is like the flame, darting here and there, blown first in one direction and then another.

Invite your mind to be the observer as you focus on your in-breath. Find the space at the top of the breath where the lungs are comfortably full and pause there for an instant, silently repeating: *I am.*

As you exhale, notice how your breath stirs the flame ever so slightly. Release all the air in your lungs, and at the bottom of the breath, pause for an instant and silently repeat: *My breath.*

I am my breath. Continue the exercise for five minutes. As you become more comfortable sitting still, gradually increase the duration of your inhalation and your exhalation.

Chapter 13

THE JOURNEY OF THE VISIONARY: RECEIVING ONE SPIRIT MEDICINE

Listen to the hidden sounds.
Use your other ears.
See the celestial sights.
Use your other eyes.
Perceive what cannot be
measured by the ordinary senses.

— FROM *PATANJALI THE SHAMAN*, ALBERTO VILLOLDO TRANSLATION

On the medicine wheel, the East is the journey of the visionary, the direction of rebirth, where the life-giving sun rises each morning, bringing us an opportunity to meet our world anew. Among indigenous people of the Americas, the East is the direction toward which the tepee and the ceremonial lodge faces, allowing the power of the new dawn to warm and fill the space.

In the East we discover that life offers us a second chance.

The East is represented by the eagle, which can soar high above the clouds, surveying the entire landscape, or home in on a mouse scurrying in the bushes. This dual perspective of both sky-level awareness and ground-level clarity is why the East is known as the way of the visionary. At this point in our journey, we learn to put the cart before the horse; to look at the possibilities before acknowledging the dour probabilities or limitations; to focus on why something can be so, rather than why it cannot.

One gift of the eagle is the ability to start afresh, free of the old stories about who we are, unbounded by expectations or fears or doubts. Every gift from Spirit entails an obligation, however, and in the East the obligation is to share the wisdom you've acquired with others. Armed with a new, more expansive map for your life, you can stop thinking your way out of one mess and into another, and appreciate each moment in all its wonder while you envision something entirely new and original that can make the world (and your world) a better place.

You know that you can transform your life at the deepest level by holding a vision of the possible. You can share this gift with others by inviting them to entertain their highest dreams, as you help them rise from their deepest nightmare. Every time a new patient walks into my office, I see the person as a healthy, luminous, and joyous being, regardless of the diagnosis they carry with them. I know that holding this healed image of my clients will help them discover their path to wellness. Only when I have this image firmly in mind do I start asking where the person is hurting and what seems to be wrong.

It's in sharing with others the healing treasures you've received that the power of these gifts becomes truly yours. It begins with healing the notion of an "I" that is separate from other beings and the cosmos, and that is powerless and helpless. If you're scared to lose your identity as an individual, you will not be able to tolerate the experience of Oneness, or the gifts of power and grace that accompany the East direction. You and I exist as separate beings only in the ordinary world.

This shift in awareness to the perspective of eagle allows you to become the dreamer instead of the dreamed. You grasp that everyone holds a piece of the cosmic puzzle, that you are not the only dreamer. You are collaborating with others and with Spirit to dream your health—and a healed and beautiful world—into being. Dreaming in this sense is going on all the time, whether or not you are aware of it. But in the journey of the visionary, you can choose to consciously participate in dreaming the world into being.

The recognition that dreaming is a collective endeavor frees you from the burden of thinking that you are the sole master of your universe but you're failing miserably at the job. At the same time, however, it allows you to own the power you *do* have to bring about change in your health and your relationships—indeed, in every aspect of your life. Armed with this awareness, you neither try to run away from crises nor are overwhelmed by them. You are able to see clearly when and how to take action, and when to let problems resolve themselves and the body heal on its own.

In the North, you learned to observe your mind during the practice of stillness. Here in the East, you come to see that the "I" that observes your experience is an inextricable part of a larger consciousness. To realize this, the Indian sage Ramana Maharshi used to recommend an exercise of self-inquiry to his students. You start by bringing your attention to the feeling of self, of *I,* and holding your attention there until the feeling of *I* disappears and only awareness remains. This is a difficult practice for most of us, so as an aid, you can begin by reflecting on the question *Who am I?,* then move on to *Who is it who is asking the question?*

This exploration will take you beyond the experience of the ego *I* to awareness of the Oneness that is the very fabric of the universe. You will come to see that your individual awareness is never truly separate from this greater consciousness; you merely experience it as separate while you have a body, a physical form. Like a wave in the sea, you are a distinct and unique individual, but at the same time you are never separate from the sea itself, from your source. Embodiment in itself is a temporary state. Your body is your local self, while the vast sea of infinite consciousness is your nonlocal self. Once you recognize your nonlocal, infinite nature, you can return to your everyday, local, embodied awareness knowing that you have the power to envision a new reality—even to grow a new body that ages and heals differently.

The journey to the East is an inner journey to the realms beyond death, where you are shown the vastness of creation. But the visionary has a duty to bring this knowledge back home. While many mystics seek to reach the heavenly realms and stay there in blissful contemplation, our intention is on creating heaven on Earth, on returning to ordinary reality to help others taste the delicious elixir of health and of Oneness. We practice healing and generosity and bring beauty to the world without any thought to what's in it for us. In fact, the opportunity to alleviate suffering is reward enough.

As it happens, there *is* a reward for the visionary, however. You will discover that you can create extraordinary health for yourself. This doesn't mean you have to instruct individual genes to switch on or off, or tell your brain what neurotransmitters to produce. You simply hold the dual eagle vision of your life—both the details and the immensity of it—and your body will do the rest. Just as stress switches on the genes that create cardiovascular disease and cancer, the serenity of eagle vision and the experience of Oneness switches on the genes for health and longevity. As eagle vision dissolves the illusion of separation, you create the spiritual conditions for health, and disease can vanish. We know that meditation results in longer telomeres, the end-caps of chromosomes that protect the integrity of DNA, and determine health and longevity.[1]

When you go on your vision quest—whether following the template laid out in Chapter 14 or some other form—you are invited to travel to a realm beyond death and retrieve your destiny from the "you" who already exists in the future. Once you encounter who you will be, you can begin to embody those qualities and attributes today. The past that stalked you will give way to a future that draws you inexorably toward who you're becoming, the self who needs no interventions or therapies or repairs. You won't have to heal what's broken—healing will happen by itself.

Rumi, in his poem "The Night Air," describes the non-doing of the person who has completed the journey of the East:

Mystics are experts at laziness. They rely on it,

Because they continuously see God working all around them.

The harvest keeps coming in, yet they

Never even did the plowing![2]

But before we can reach the point of non-doing, there is work to be done. The path of the eagle is not for someone looking for a quick route to a happy life. The story of Siddhartha, the Indian prince who became the Buddha, illustrates the journey of the eagle: the awakening of vision, the call to destiny, and the return to the world to share what we've learned.

Siddhartha: The Gifts of One Spirit Medicine

According to legend, the Buddha was born a prince, Siddhartha—whose name means "all wishes fulfilled." His father was a great king who was determined to keep his son from experiencing the anxiety and pain of the world. He was the ultimate helicopter parent, sheltering young Siddhartha from all ugliness. The prince grew up surrounded by flowering gardens and attended by servants who catered to his every need, oblivious to what was happening outside the palace walls where the commoners lived. Like Siddhartha, we want to live in a bubble of happiness and comfort, in a gated community removed from anything that might cause us distress. His father represents our tendency to isolate ourselves, to build our own little palace in the middle of the slums and focus on our own needs, oblivious to the discomfort of others.

But human beings are social animals, attuned to one another's cues, empathizing with one another's pain and wired to experience sadness at the sight of someone else's suffering. One day, after Siddhartha had left childhood behind, he became curious about what went on outside the palace. Against his father's wishes, he asked his charioteer to drive him around the countryside so he could see the people he would rule one day and understand how they lived. For Siddhartha to mature, he had to break out of the psychic bubble of his childhood.

As he rode in his regal chariot, Siddhartha came upon four sights that unsettled him deeply. The first was an old man, hobbling along on the side of the road, groaning in pain. "Why is he groaning?" Siddhartha asked his driver. The driver replied, "Because he is old and infirm, so he suffers."

This was a huge wake-up call for Siddhartha, who had never imagined such things as aging and infirmity. He had heard of suffering but didn't believe it existed, yet here it was right in front of him. "Will I grow old and become infirm?" he asked. "Yes," his driver said.

Wealthy, well fed, and groomed to rule the entire kingdom from his cocoon of luxury, Siddhartha wasn't in any pain, but his response to seeing someone else suffer was to ask, *What about me?* Later, after he became a Buddha, he turned this worry into compassion for others, no longer focusing on his own vulnerability. We are all responsible for our own well-being, but that's very different from "looking out for number one" and putting our needs ahead of everyone else's.

It's no accident that the first suffering Siddhartha encountered was a man who was soon to leave behind his old life and experience death. Siddhartha was leaving behind his old life of comfort and entering into an unfamiliar realm: *How long will I live? How long can I avoid infirmity? Who am I, if not a prince so powerful that I will live forever, happy all the time?* It pained him to discover there was nothing he could do to restore the old man's youth and vitality. *So much for being the all-powerful ruler of the land,* Siddhartha thought. He had to discard that role, he realized.

The first sight on the road corresponds to the First Noble Truth of Buddhism: In life, there is suffering. This is the truth we come to accept when we do the work of the South on the medicine wheel, shedding outmoded roles and victim identities to give birth to a nobler role as the author of our own destiny.

Siddhartha was still wondering if death was a long way off when he saw another sight that distressed him: a naked man by the side of the road, begging for coins or food. "Driver," Siddhartha asked, "what's wrong with that man?"

Siddhartha's driver replied, "That's a hungry, diseased beggar." And then Siddhartha asked, "Might I be like that beggar someday?" "Yes," said the driver, "because even though you're rich and will rule over the entire land, you won't have the power to avoid disease. You, too, will grow old, and lose your health and beauty."

Siddhartha was shocked. He had no idea there would ever be an end to his robust good health or his ability to realize his desires, but now he was hearing that such an outcome was inevitable. *There must be a mistake,* he thought. *This might happen to others, but could it really happen to me?* We all want to believe that bad things and growing old only happen to other people. When we are young we learn that people grow old and die, but we never believe that will happen to us.

Siddhartha's revelation at the sight of the beggar corresponds to the Second Noble Truth: Suffering is caused by attachment. Our happiness depends on having what we want and not having what we don't want. When we're content, we don't want anything to change. Instead of realizing that change is inevitable, and looking forward to what else might come along and delight us, we cling to the old, until our closets are filled with old clothing, our basements with old stuff, and our minds with old thoughts and beliefs. Sometimes we even become attached to a bad situation—an abusive marriage or a terrible job—thinking, *It's probably better than being single at 50 or not having any work.* Afraid of uncertainty, we cling to old roles and identities, even though they no longer fit. But the way forward is to let go of our old roles and attachments—to release them into the fire, as we did in the journey of the healer. We have to die to our old notions and let our expectations change as we go forth into the unknown.

When I received my diagnosis of "you should be dead," my long list of what I needed to be happy was suddenly wiped clean. The only things that mattered were my health and, if that couldn't be restored, preparing to die. Today, I purposely keep my happiness list very short, with those two items at the very top.

We're attached not only to what's in the past—what we've outgrown but still keep in our closets—but also to what the future may bring. We cling to the idea that life will get better. The notion that something unpleasant might await makes us freeze in fear. The diseased man whom Siddhartha encounters represents our primal survival fears: not having enough food, money, health, or power. The old man is the future we dread and attempt to avoid at all costs. But when we face our fear of death in the journey of the jaguar and learn to walk through the jungle of uncertainty, we cease to cower helplessly in terror at the unknown.

Siddhartha, however, was still unnerved by the possibility of his own sickness and decline when he came across a third distressing sight alongside the road: a corpse.

"What's wrong with him? Why isn't he getting up and going about his business?" Siddhartha asked his driver. "He's dead," said the driver.

"There's no way to bring him back to life?" Siddhartha asked. "Alas, no," came the answer.

Siddhartha was deeply saddened. "Will my life also end someday?" Indeed, the driver told him; death is inevitable for all.

The corpse alongside the road corresponds to the Third Noble Truth: To end suffering, we have to release all attachments, even the attachment to life itself. We have to stop grasping at what is slipping away from us, or yearning for what we've lost and can't seem to regain. And we have to stop believing that inner peace comes only when our wishes come true.

Upon hearing that he, too, would someday die, Siddhartha was very upset. But there was one last sight that would shake his awareness: a sadhu, or holy man, sitting cross-legged in meditation beside the road. The man seemed utterly tranquil, beyond all fear and suffering. Siddhartha asked his driver to stop the carriage, and he hurriedly approached the sadhu to ask how he had achieved such serenity.

"You, too, can transcend suffering and death," promised the sadhu. "You need only sit still under that tree over there, refusing all food and drink, until you know that you are free from the death that is stalking you."

Siddhartha returned to the palace but found that life as he knew it had lost its appeal. The sadhu's words never left him. A few years later, he abandoned his life of riches and ease and, drawn toward his destiny, set out as a wandering monk to find an end to his suffering. Once the veil is lifted and, like Siddhartha, we have a glimpse of suffering—the world's and our own—our old ways begin to chafe, and the quest for healing begins. How long or how fraught with challenges the journey of the visionary will be varies with the individual. But by now you have a pretty good idea that the road is steep and seldom straight, and that healing involves dedicated physical, mental, and emotional preparation.

Siddhartha spent six years in deep meditation, with little sustenance for his body, but still he was unable to find the answers he sought. Finally, in an act of desperation and surrender, he sat down under a fig tree and vowed not to move until he had discovered the cause of suffering and how to end to it. Children played around him, dogs barked, young women tried to seduce or distract him, and robbers took his monk's bag with his few possessions. But Siddhartha simply sat there, turning his gaze within, studying the nature of his own mind. He opened his heart and released any expectations about what would happen. And then, according to legend, after a harrowing night, at daybreak he experienced enlightenment under what was thereafter known as the Bodhi Tree. (*Bodhi* means "awakened.") Later the Buddha described what he had awakened to:

I came to direct knowledge of aging and death, direct knowl-edge of the origination of aging and death, direct knowledge of the cessation of aging and death, direct knowledge of the path leading to the cessation of aging and death . . .[3]

Whether we call it enlightenment, realization, or Oneness, the experience that transformed Siddhartha into the Buddha, the Awakened One, was profoundly healing and, at the same time, disarmingly simple. "The truth of cessation is a personal discovery," the Tibetan Buddhist teacher Chögyam Trungpa Rinpoche said. "It is not mystical and it does not have any connotations of religion or psychology, it is simply your experience . . ."[4]

Siddhartha had set out to heal his own suffering, and from his quest he brought back to humanity the means to end their suffering in the face of disease, old age, and death. This is the gift of the eagle, the fruit of the journey of the visionary.

One Spirit Medicine Revealed

In the direction of the East on the medicine wheel, you lose yourself to find yourself. Having died to the old, you are reborn into a new life. You realize that the temporal you who dwells in the physical world is ever-changing, but the timeless you is unchanging and never suffers. The timeless you is never ill and will never die. This realization can help you return to perfect health and guide every cell in your system to grow a new body more suitable for itself.

We began our discovery of the timeless self in the South, where we shed our old roles and preconceived notions about who we really are and, like Parsifal, healed the wounded masculine within us. We continued the journey in the West, with Psyche teaching us that we had to cross a threshold into the unknown if we were going to free ourselves from the prison of our own fear, most notably our fear of death, and retrieve the gifts of the goddess, of realizing our immortality. Having accomplished that, we went to the North, where we learned to be still and focus inward, drawing on the collective wisdom of those who have gone before us. The splendor of the cosmos was revealed to us, just as it was to Arjuna.

When we reached the East, all the steps on the path, all the trials we endured, suddenly made sense. Opening to a wider perspective, we grasped the paradox of our existence: that each of us is both infinitesimal, a mere speck, and infinitely vast, simultaneously nothing and everything. Even enlightenment, we discovered, has a nothing-special, everyday side to it. And we learned that like Siddhartha, once we experience Oneness, we can bring that wisdom to the world.

So, while you may intellectually grasp the lessons associated with the four directions on the medicine wheel, it is only with the direct experience of Oneness that these principles take hold and shift your life. In the East, we have to confront our inner demons much as the Buddha—and Jesus—did. Jesus did not wrestle his demons to the ground; he simply told them firmly to be on their way. The Buddha, rather than fight his demons, fed them: "Here, you want my head, take it. You want my body, take it." His timeless self understood that he was not his body or his head, and when he failed to engage with his tormentors, they became bored and left. The great temptation for us is to battle our demons, thinking we can emerge victorious. And then 30 years later, scratched and bloodied, we finally recognize the futility of battle. Our terrible relationship with our mother, our father, or our ex is still there. Our children are still angry with us. The lessons of the East and the way of the visionary give us a better way to move our demons along.

Even when we've received the gifts of Spirit, we still have to meet the challenges of our physical existence. And awakening doesn't absolve us of the need to refine our thinking and continually improve our attitudes and behavior. I like to think that the Eastern traditions are all about waking up, while the Western ones are about growing up. Both are equally important. We are not looking for the sense of Oneness that babies share, but what we can experience as mature adults. In fact, there is nothing as boring as the immature babble we too often confuse for spirituality in America.

Even the Dalai Lama feels anger, he admits; despite his qualities, he's only human. But he doesn't feed this anger or act upon it, so it quickly passes. He approaches life with compassion and eagle vision: "I always look at any event from a wider angle," His Holiness told a *Time* interviewer.[5] Jesus came back from the desert with the wisdom teachings of *Love your neighbor as yourself* and *Turn the other cheek*, but he did a lot of walking, teaching, and maturing before his work was done. The Buddha, after his enlightenment, didn't retreat to a mountaintop to dwell in bliss. For the next 45 years, he was very much in the world, helping others awaken and heal.

If the Eastern traditions are about waking up, and the Western ones about growing up, the way of the shaman is about *showing up* for your life and for others. It is about living courageously and becoming accountable.

So how will *your* life be different after your journey through the medicine wheel? For one thing, the perspective of eagle vision will help you navigate your life with greater freedom. The work you do will seem natural, consonant with your talents and values. And the healing of body, mind, and spirit you experience will have such force behind it that you will feel compelled to serve the world however you can.

With that foretaste of what the journey of the visionary will bring, we can take the last step in the journey: the vision quest.

Chapter 14

THE VISION QUEST

How do you apply quantum mechanics to everyday life? . . .
Does quantum theory teach you how to walk on the Earth?
How to change the weather?
How to identify yourself with the creative principle,
with Nature, with the Divine?
Does it teach you how to live every moment of your life
as an act of power?

— From *Dance of the Four Winds*, by Alberto Villoldo and Erik Jendresen

It's one thing to read about growing a new body and another to experience it. Just as reading about Siddhartha's enlightenment is not enough to free you from disease, old age, and death, reading this book will give you information but not wisdom. The final and most important practice for attaining it is the diet, the supplements, your journey through the medicine wheel, and the vision quest.

The vision quest can heal your body and mend your soul. Like Parsifal, you must search for the Holy Grail. Like Psyche, you must return from the underworld with the elixir of immortality.

Like Arjuna, you must discover the secrets of the cosmos. And like Siddhartha, you must leave the comfort of the castle or the couch and sit under your version of the Bodhi Tree.

Think of it as a kind of spiritual health prevention. Don't wait until you are sick to explore the benefits of the diet, or until the end of your life to explore the journey beyond death.

We all have a dozen reasons for why we can't leave the castle or the couch just yet: not enough money, not enough time, too many e-mails to respond to. I myself postponed the journey until I received a diagnosis and saw the end of my life before me. My advice? Don't wait until then!

Ideally, you will make your vision quest in a natural setting, sitting with the elements—rain, wind, sun, heat, cold—and putting your body under mild physiological stress by intermittent fasting. However, the purpose of a vision quest is not to rough it without food or water but to discover in the wilderness that you are a citizen of the earth. Your fast will awaken the body's self-repair systems and stimulate production of stem cells in the brain and every organ in your body. Your time in nature will reveal to you how the experience of Oneness is available to you at all times.

Unless you upgrade your brain first, however, the vision quest will be nothing more than a camping trip. But after you detox and then power your brain with superfoods during the Grow a New Body program, the quest can be a face-to-face meeting with your destiny. If you have applied yourself diligently to the practices suggested throughout the book, you will taste the Oneness of creation as you continue to grow a new body. Remember that the body is the vessel for the spirit. Your flesh and bones and cells and neurons will follow the lead of the spirit to become a resilient and vibrant vessel for it to reside in during its brief journey here on the earth.

Taking the Challenge

"What do you mean, a vision quest?" Sally, an inveterate New Yorker, demanded. "You know I don't rough it, and this means I don't go anywhere without room service!" A city girl inside and out, Sally was a high-powered editor at a women's fashion magazine. She wanted no part of being in the wilderness alone for three days, subsisting on nothing but water.

"But do you want to be miserable for the rest of your life?" I asked her. "Wouldn't it be better to be miserable for three days and get it over with, so you can have a new life? Besides," I added slyly, "there's probably a good magazine article in there as well."

Reluctantly, Sally agreed to do a vision quest, and I dropped her off in a canyon surrounded by steep cliffs in the red rocks of southern Utah. She had plenty of water and a good tent and a sleeping bag. I did not explain to her that although nature is the preferred setting for a vision quest, in fact you could do one anywhere, even in the middle of New York City. The point is to disconnect from the technologically wired world and discard the belief that if you aren't continually checking your e-mail and social media, your life will fall apart. I also instructed Sally to pray.

"But I don't know how to pray," she protested.

"Give thanks to the Creator," I told her. "And if that doesn't work," I said offhandedly as I drove off, "pray that the wolves won't get you." There were no wolves in the area, but Sally got my point. We can find our way to Spirit through prayer or meditation, but if we get caught up in exactly *how* we're supposed to pray or communicate with Spirit, we'll remain closed to the wisdom we might receive.

Sally was a longtime client. Rich and smart, she had been a beauty in her 20s, and even in her mid-50s was undeniably glamorous. She was also hyperkinetic, used to getting her own way, and cursed with the worst luck in relationships of anyone I've ever met. Sally was taking Ritalin during the day to manage her ADHD, and trazodone, a powerful antidepressant and anti-anxiety drug, to help her sleep at night. She kept bouncing from one abusive relationship to the next, to the point where she had become so desensitized that she preferred, as she put it, "to use men as toys." But she also admitted she could not get rid of those toys without a lot of heartache.

The vision quest challenged many of Sally's city-comfort habits. There was no gourmet grocery store nearby. She could not switch on the news, and there was no Internet. She hated the thought of being in the wild by herself. But she could not bear the idea of continuing her life of romantic wretchedness and pharmaceutical misery.

"I loved peeing in the woods," Sally told me with a grin when I picked her up at the end of the three days. Her hair was disheveled and her face full of grime, but somehow her clothing was impeccable. I wondered how she had managed that. Then she admitted she had brought a clean outfit for each day. (Some habits die hard.) The retreat had not been easy for her, she said. On day one she tried calling a car service to come and get her, but there was no cell phone connection. At night, she was convinced she would be food for the wolves and imagined them circling her tent. She prayed for dawn to arrive. But by the second evening, she began to enjoy watching the stars from inside her sleeping bag, which she dragged out of the tent when she realized she wasn't going to attract a pack of hungry predators. Sally had never seen so many stars in the sky—in fact, had not seen stars at all for years, since the city lights of New York make it hard to see anything in the night sky. Hunger pangs kept her awake the first evening, but after that she slept like a baby. And then there were the lights. "During the first night I felt like I was camping in a parking lot," she said. "There were headlights shining into the tent, so bright that they woke me up. But when I went outside, it was perfectly dark, except for the stars." At first Sally thought extraterrestrials had been shining the lights, but then she realized that in her dreams she was being shown "the light."

Sally came back from her vision quest with a deep appreciation for nature and for how precious her life—indeed, all life—is. She also decided to take a hiatus from men. She began to see her immediate attraction to certain men as a warning sign that they weren't the kind who would be good to her. Then six months after her vision quest, she started dating a quiet, gentle man—a "really soft man," in her words. But the most notable change after her vision quest was that Sally's ADHD mysteriously went away. As she remained on a gluten-free, dairy-free diet, incorporating healthy vegetables, lots of omega-3 oils, and a low-protein diet, her hyperactivity and moodiness dissipated, and she no longer required Ritalin to function during the day or trazodone to sleep at night.

The Bread Maker

When Samuel came to see me, he weighed 260 pounds. He ate almost nothing but bread, pasta, and processed foods, and he had high blood pressure, elevated cholesterol, and insulin resistance. Samuel was a publisher whose list included books on health, raw foods, and healthy diets, yet he was a compulsive eater. Addicted to processed carbs, Samuel was suffering from *diabesity*—diabetes associated with obesity. It's the new epidemic of the civilized world. I mentioned to Samuel that incidences of type 1 diabetes, in which the pancreas is unable to produce any insulin, had dropped 60 percent during World War II as a result of food scarcity. I told him that fasting during his vision quest would give him the same benefit, without starving him for more than a few days.[1]

Samuel had tried every diet plan in the world and at that point was following the Paleo diet. As I described in Chapter 5, the Paleo diet is based on what preagricultural, Paleolithic-era humans ate. Hunter-gatherers, they subsisted mostly on greens and the occasional small game or fish. There are no essential carbs, I explained to him, but there are essential proteins and fatty acids, and we could live the rest of our lives without ever eating another piece of toast. But Samuel was eating way too much protein. I suggested that Samuel cut down his intake and also stay away from red meat—beef and pork—which the ancient hunter-gatherers rarely ate. "It's fine to have an occasional steak," I told Samuel. "But when you do, be sure it's grass fed and free-range, not from animals that were grain fed or pumped full of antibiotics. Fish, if they are pan-sized and come from clean water and contain no mercury, are great. But the bread and pasta have to go."

While many people embrace the Paleo diet, they forget to embrace the Paleolithic beliefs about the Oneness of all life, the communion with nature and Spirit. "Those beliefs are a big part of creating health in your body," I told Samuel. "The diet alone doesn't work without Spirit being enlisted to help you change your health."

Samuel was a tough cookie. He assured me he would put away his bread-making machine, but his cupboards were filled with canned foods, most of which contained sugar and gluten. And Samuel's systemic inflammation was being caused by gluten and dairy, which were destroying his gut flora. Samuel wasn't going to give up easily.

So one afternoon we went to his apartment, and I started emptying his cupboards, tossing out canned foods, wheat flour that was stored in the closet next to the bread-making machine, and the bread-making machine itself. He even had toothpaste that contained sugar! As I was taking it all out to the garbage chute, I could tell that Samuel was distraught. He loved his bread machine, and deep in his mind he believed he simply had to put it away for a brief hiatus. But here I was recycling his beloved contraption!

When we're young, our mothers give us food to comfort us, so from then on when we feel stressed we tend to gravitate to comfort foods—the sugary treats we grew up on. The result is that over the decades, the marvelous flora in our guts become addicted to sugars, carbs, and nasty fats, so when we fast for more than 12 hours, the Candida go into revolt. *We're* not starving, but *they* are, so they begin releasing chemical toxins that signal starvation to the brain. Even though we don't actually need nourishment, we become ravenously hungry, simply because the yeast want to feed.

The gut microbes are extraordinarily smart, however, and they learn very quickly. In just 24 hours, we can break their food addictions and begin to establish a new balance in the colony, allowing good flora to flourish. Cutting off sugars, starches, and harmful fats, taking *S. boulardii* and quality probiotics allows the good bugs to recolonize your gut. That's why very short bouts of fasting are so important: they restore the balance in the gut and turn on all the body's repair systems.

Samuel knew intellectually that processed carbs like bread and pasta are extremely addictive, stimulating the same reward centers in the brain that cocaine does. He had badly damaged his gut with all the gluten and processed food he had been consuming for years, but that wasn't enough to convince him to make the changes necessary to heal his body and reclaim his life. That day by the garbage chute, we almost had a fistfight. It was the first time since high school that someone had shoved me against a wall!

What happened next was miraculous. Within four days, Samuel began to feel better and lose weight—more than a pound a day. And he was doing it by eliminating gluten, wheat, carbs, dairy, and sugars from his diet, and taking the supplements I recommended in Chapter 6. It wasn't easy. A couple of times he called me during the night crying, as images from his unhappy childhood and adolescence kept flooding his mind. By the end of the week, however, Samuel had lost close to 10 pounds, and his brain fog had cleared. He was sleeping soundly for the first time in decades. And the supplements were helping him eliminate the toxins previously stored in his fat, preventing them from being reabsorbed by his gut. Samuel was ready for the vision quest.

While God seems to prefer churches, Spirit seems to prefer wild places. In fact, nearly all the memorable encounters with the divine recorded in myth and history have occurred in a natural setting—the wilderness, a mountaintop, the desert—but seldom inside a cathedral. Samuel decided he would do his vision quest at the Fairchild Tropical Botanic Garden in Coral

Gables, Florida, near his summer home. He would go to the Gardens at seven every morning when the park opened and remain on the grounds until it closed. His task was to speak to no one and simply to sit in the shade of the trees he enjoyed most and drink lots of water throughout the day.

After his three-day vision quest, Samuel told me, "While I didn't meet God, I discovered a quiet that I had known only as a child. After the second day, my mind stopped thinking about all the important things I had to do. I'd always felt that if I didn't do all those things, the world would end. The tropical trees showed me that I was like them—shedding leaves, budding with new growth, needing deep roots to hold me up during the high winds and storms—and that it was my job to help create a world that was not ruined by human folly and greed.

"The most difficult part was the grumbling in my stomach," he said. "For the first time in my life, I experienced real hunger. At first, all I could think about was a chocolate bar I had in my car. But after day two, my obsession with feeling hungry passed. After day three, I think I could have gone without food for another week. The physical discomfort of not eating was gone, and I felt tremendous energy. My head was clear and lucid, and I felt a tremendous sense of peace."

I continued working with Samuel for another year, and he remained free of wheat and dairy. He had rescued his bread machine from the garbage chute, but he never brought it out again, and after six months, his blood sugar levels returned to normal. We did regular blood tests of IGF-1, a tumor marker, and found that his levels decreased by more than 30 percent.

During his vision quest, he discovered an inner life he had read about in the books he published but had never been entirely convinced was real. Because of his meditation practice, he now explores his inner world with the same sense of adventure that early explorers must have felt as they discovered new lands in the Americas. He is fascinated by the joyous landscapes of his mind, which he is finally able to access, instead of ruminating on his to-do list and regrets about his childhood.

Returning to Life

George, a physician, was literally dragged into my office by his wife. He was going through a very aggressive chemotherapy that was not producing the desired results. His tumor markers were not budging, and his immune system was suppressed. He had agreed to see me only because his wife, a student at our Light Body School, had pointed out that he had nothing left to lose.

George did not see the relationship between his stressful job, his caffeine intake—half a dozen cups of coffee a day—his carb-heavy diet, and his cancer.

My friend doctor Dean Ornish, at the University of California Medical Center, discovered that patients with prostate cancer who switched to a primarily plant-based, low-calorie diet could dramatically reverse early-stage cancers within a six-month period.[2] It's amazing the power that green plants have to switch on the genes that create health and switch off the genes that create disease. I immediately asked George to go on a plant-based diet rich in cruciferous vegetables, including broccoli and Brussels sprouts, and healthy fats like avocados and walnuts. He was to begin each morning with a detoxifying green juice. I asked him to steer clear of gluten and all grains and to avoid red meat.

After decades of eating the toxic fast-food fare in the hospital, in just three weeks, George lost nearly 10 pounds. He was feeling better every day, and the tumor markers were beginning to recede.

"Now we have to do your vision quest," I told him. The last time George had been out in nature, he said, was as a Boy Scout 40 years earlier. When he wasn't working in the hospital, he spent all his quality time with his children, so he didn't feel he should take a weekend to go into the wild alone.

"I'll do my vision quest in the hospital, while I'm working," he decided. "I might be a little fog-brained at first, but that's not a problem. When an emergency case comes through, the adrenaline allows me to shake off any mental fog right away."

George's hospital was a trauma center in Miami, and I asked him to say a prayer for each patient he treated. And I suggested that while he was patching them up, he should admire the beauty of the blood vessels, muscles, and other tissues that make up the body. I also told him to be mindful of seeing each of his patients as a human being, not as a gunshot wound. Of all the things I asked him to do, he said this was the hardest, because like most doctors, he had been trained to view patients impersonally, maintaining professional distance. Most doctors, afraid perhaps of being overwhelmed by their feelings in the face of great suffering, are more comfortable relating to symptoms and organs than to living, breathing, terrified patients.

"Understand that you are doing Spirit's work every time you touch someone," I told him.

Whatever your profession, once you understand that Spirit's work can become *your* work—that Spirit can work through your hands, your heart, your feelings, your skills—your life acquires greater meaning. George told me that the wildest time in the ER seems to be during the summer full moon, when the number of patients coming in with gunshot wounds, injuries from accidents, or drug and alcohol overdoses appears to be greater than at any other time of the year. George began his vision quest during a full moon and decided he would practice monitoring his breath to remain mindful of what he was experiencing and to connect with each patient as a human being rather than as "the gunshot wound in Bed 6." He tried to note each inhalation and exhalation, and in the moment of stillness between breaths, he would pause, appreciating every precious drop of air.

"I can do without the food," George told me, "but I know that I can't do without the coffee." I enjoy coffee myself, and I could understand George's predicament. In fact, coffee is used as a sacred medicine in many parts of the world. The Sufi whirling dervishes are notorious coffee drinkers. And coffee, perhaps more than any other food, is a powerful activator of Nrf2 detox pathways and longevity proteins in the body. No one knows exactly how or why this works, but even oncologists today are recommending that liver cancer patients drink three to four cups of the black stuff each day. But if you're stressed-out and living in a constant state of fight-or-flight, too much caffeine only exacerbates the problem. I explained to George that it was essential that he cut back on drinking coffee at least a week before his vision quest began. He needed to give his frayed nervous system a much-needed rest. For George, the issue was that his brain was awash in cortisol caused by the caffeine.

When I saw George at my office two weeks after his week-long vision quest, he was exhilarated. He had given up coffee, cheating only twice with an espresso at the start of the week. The first day of fasting, he felt incredibly weak and hungry. But he concentrated on seeing every patient, no matter how broken, as an angel in the making. He found himself touching people he would never before have come near, except with latex gloves and an air of detachment: a homeless man drenched in his own urine, a thug with a bullet in his leg. By day three, George had tapped into an extraordinary reservoir of energy. His hunger pangs had dissipated, he was drinking a lot of water, and he was amazed at how much he was defecating every day, given that he was eating no food whatsoever. His body was cleansing and detoxing, eliminating decades of waste that had built up inside every cell of his body.

By day three, George had changed over to burning fats instead of sugars to fuel his body and brain. As his higher brain switched on, he was able to envision a life of health and well-being for himself. And from his newfound vantage point, he redefined his work. He was no longer a mechanic fixing arms and stomachs and broken bones; he was an artist helping people return to health from the brink of death. Last time I spoke with George, his cancer was in remission. He has recovered his life.

Communion with Creation

One Spirit Medicine is what the shamans call the experience of Oneness that allows you to understand the workings of creation. This understanding is not academic or intellectual; it's experiential and sensory—a *knowingness* that pervades every cell of your body. You don't suddenly have a eureka moment and apprehend the first law of thermodynamics and the conservation of energy. Instead, you experience a transcendent awareness that penetrates your whole being. You truly grasp that energy and consciousness can never be destroyed, only transformed into myriad shapes and forms, one of which happens to be you.

Each of my clients mentioned in this chapter—Sally, Samuel, and George—experienced a deep, intuitive understanding of the wonder of Oneness. For Sally, this happened as she lay in the desert under the night sky, watching the stars that she knew had always been there, hidden behind the light pollution of New York City. For Samuel, observing his hunger and cravings, and realizing how much he loved to grapple with profound issues, led him to a deeper exploration of his mind. He began by defining a problem, any problem, and then asking himself, *Who is it who is thinking about this? Who is it who is asking the question?* Those questions eventually led him to Zen, a meditation practice stripped of all adornment, in which the practitioner simply observes his breath and witnesses the mind in all its madness and creativity. As for George, he learned that he could see Spirit in everyone and, indeed, *needed* to see Spirit in everyone in order to become a better doctor and healer. In the process, he healed himself.

Each of these individuals came back to see me several more times, even when there was nothing wrong, nothing that had to be repaired. They wanted more of the medicine that had healed them physically and emotionally.

Normally, healing the spirit is the last step for people seeking healing in our society, but it's the first step for those seeking to grow a new body. The vision quest that Sally, Samuel, and George each undertook—returning to the wild alone, with only water to sustain them—was the same sort of retreat, the same sort of quest for Spirit, that Jesus and the Buddha undertook. They confronted the demons of hunger, anger, and self-judgment. Their vision quests repaired their bodies and primed their brains for their great missions. They returned home afterward with a newfound sense of purpose, and a mission to share what they'd learned with humanity.

During a second vision quest, Sally had a dream that answered a central question: *What is the theme for the next stage of my life?* I had previously explained to her that you can't solve problems in your dreams with your sugar brain, but with her brain properly healed, she was able to access uncommon wisdom. Here's the dream as she related it to me:

I'm in the past, centuries ago, and I tell my beloved I'll find him again and not to worry. I go through a glass door—it is our time to say good-bye—and suddenly, I'm in a museum, in the present. I'm amazed by my modern clothing. A man is there with me. I realize I must look for my beloved here and wonder, Is it this man? He turns and tells me that he is not the one I am looking for, but he will take me to the one I am seeking. I am searching for the Beloved—not the human beloved, but Spirit. And Spirit is already walking by my side.

"In the dream there was deep familiarity," Sally said, "as if my beloved had always been there. And I felt that in a previous lifetime I had also been searching for God." She realized that she was not only looking for the right partner but also searching for Spirit, the only lover who would truly fulfill her. She understood that she had to find Spirit *in* her partner and together *with* her partner.

Power Animals

In ancient cultures, when you did a vision quest, a power animal would appear to you in a dream or waking vision—and you might have this experience, too. The word *animal* comes from the same root as *anima,* Latin for soul, breath, the life force. Carl Jung used *anima* to refer to the feminine principle. An animal, then, is an expression of the feminine aspect of the soul of the world. The power animal symbolizes the wild, undomesticated aspect of your being, the aspect that has no boss, isn't wedded to a laundry list, and is free as the wind. The power animal represents your unfettered soul, the part of you that hasn't been beaten down by the modern world.

If you visit certain caves in France and Spain, you can see ancient paintings of bears, bison, wolves, and other animals depicted by Paleolithic artists. The grace, power, dignity, and beauty of these creatures comes through with great intensity. The painting of "The Sorcerer" in the Trois-Frères cave in Ariège, France, depicts a mythic figure, part human and part stag. Creatures that are part human and part animal represent our kinship with all animals.

To the humans of the Paleolithic period, animals were sacred. Today in the West, only pets are sacred, and many people eat meat from animals raised in the most inhumane ways and butchered in slaughterhouses before being shrink-wrapped and sent to grocery stores. Humanity has a collective memory of our association with animals, however, and we see this in Native American cultures, where kinship is based on clans named for their totems: wolf, bear, rattlesnake, and the like. But those of us living in cities have little to no relationship with power animals of any kind.

Most of us would be hard-pressed even to name our state or national animal. Every U.S. state has a symbolic animal, like California's grizzly bear and Colorado's bighorn sheep. Similarly, countries have symbolic animals. The rooster is associated with France, the bear with Russia, and the panda with China. The eagle is the national symbol of at least eight countries, including the United States. Nowadays, we are so detached from nature that we would probably come up with state or national symbols representing favorite social media apps!

When you connect with a power animal, you are in effect connecting with the psyche or soul of nature. During your vision quest, you will invite a power animal to come to you and teach you its ways. You do this by simply stating your intention in the form of a prayer. For example: *Great Spirit, creator of all, bless me with a visit from one of your creatures that will bring me the wisdom and strength I need in my life at this time.*

When you first encounter a Spirit animal, you may have no idea why that particular creature has come to you. Just accept its presence and remember that the power animal is an emissary from Spirit, come to guide you in taking the next step in your development. Power animals are protectors and teachers.

Sally brought a wolf back from her vision quest—the very animal she was most afraid would make a meal of her. When I asked her what the wolf symbolized to her, she said she felt it had come to teach her about belonging to a pack. The wolf ranges far, traveling alone, but always returns home to its mate. And wolves mate for life, or at least practice serial monogamy, which is a lesson Sally very much wanted to learn, once she found the right partner.

On his vision quest, Samuel encountered a squirrel in a dream; it offered him an acorn and then snatched it back, scratching Samuel's face in the process. His dream befuddled both of us for a while, until I asked Samuel to hold a dialogue with this power animal. I asked Samuel to draw a line down the center of a sheet of paper and write his name on the left side, and then sketch the shape of the power animal on the right side of the page.

In this method of dialoguing with a power animal, you start by asking the power animal, "Who are you?" Then you listen for a response and write down what the power animal says. Samuel's squirrel was clear that it had come to teach him not to hoard things. One of the first things the squirrel said was that it knew exactly how many acorns it needed to support it through the long winter and that more acorns would not mean more safety or security. Samuel understood that the acorns referred to his weight. He didn't need to store any more body fat for the long winter that would never come. And then he saw that his hoarding habit had been passed down to him through three generations of ancestors who had been persecuted, stripped of their possessions and property, and then forced to flee their countries. It was a defining moment for Samuel when he realized that he no longer needed to continue living the familial story of scarcity. The squirrel had come to teach him to spend more time scurrying through the trees and soaring as he jumped between branches, and less time storing food for the lean years.

When you retrieve a power animal during a vision quest, you are inviting into your life the qualities it represents. Through the animal, you can explore new facets of yourself. You can cultivate a relationship with a power animal by embodying it—by imagining that you are looking with the eyes of a jaguar, say, or bounding gracefully like a gazelle. Or you could do yoga or one of the martial arts that have postures or movements named for the animals they suggest. Think of yoga poses like camel, cobra, lion, and downward-facing dog, or tai chi moves with evocative names like Birds Returning to the Trees at Dusk, Dragon Sweeping Tail, and Heavenly Horse Flying Across the Sky, or the five styles of kung fu: tiger, leopard, crane, snake, and dragon.

Spend time dialoguing with your power animal whenever you can. Let it teach you how to walk softly on the earth and how to see things that are not obvious to human eyes. Its power awakens your primordial instincts, which can serve you in all situations.

A Life-Changing Experience

A vision quest can change your life forever. It's impossible to forget the intense awakening to your luminous nature that comes as the hunger pangs subside. This awakening lifts the veil between the visible and invisible worlds. With the veil lifted, you instantly become aware of your Oneness with Spirit and all creation.

The vision quest takes a commitment, and it will most likely cause you some physical and emotional discomfort. But it's a powerful way to begin your transformation, a means of jump-starting your personal evolution and your new body.

Creating Your Own Three-Day Vision Quest

The vision quest takes place in a natural setting. Fasting and meditation are the central practices to bring about the deep ketosis necessary to trigger the rapid repair and growth of a new body, and a profound experience of Oneness with all creation.

Before beginning a vision quest, be sure you have been following the 18-hour daily fast described in Chapter 5 for at least three months. This will ensure that your body knows how to switch from burning glucose to burning fat as its energy source. Otherwise you will just be hungry and miserable in the wilderness for three days without deriving the benefits of the vision quest. It will also give your body time to eliminate toxins and upgrade your brain.

The following suggestions will help make your three-day vision quest a success:

Location: To find a suitable location for the vision quest, imagine you are being led by a jaguar to a secluded spot in nature. Cats have an uncanny sense of where to lie, while dogs are always sniffing around, trying one spot and then another. Your imaginary cat will lead you true. Be sure the place is beautiful, safe, and sufficiently secluded that you will not be interrupted by hikers.

If you choose not to go into the wilderness for your vision quest, you can pick a place closer to home—even in an urban area. The stories of Samuel and George in this chapter offer ideas on choosing an alternative location.

Equipment: You can bring a sleeping bag and sleeping pad, and, if you wish, a tent. Be sure to pack a notebook or journal and a pen, so you can record your dreams and any memories or strong feelings that arise. Do *not* bring a computer or other electronic devices, or any reading material. If there are tasks you must accomplish, do them mindfully, as George did, reminding yourself that Spirit is present.

You can bring a cell phone but only to use in case of emergency. Be sure to inform a friend or family member (or if you're staying in a public park or preserve, a ranger) exactly where you're going to be. If you wish, you can ask someone to check on you once a day, preferably in the evening, as long as they don't distract you.

Setting the space: When you arrive at the spot for your vision quest, draw a circle about 20 feet in diameter around your tent. This is your spot, and you will stay inside this circle for the next three days, stepping out only to relieve yourself in the woods or behind a bush. (Pack a few plastic garbage bags for collecting waste that you will dispose of when you leave.)

Fasting: Fasting is a central part of the vision quest. In addition to bringing the body into deep ketosis, it turns on production of stem cells in the brain and all organs of the body.

You will get hungry, and your stomach will start growling. Often, the growling will be louder in your head than in your stomach; your limbic brain misses glucose-rich food and believes it will die if it skips a meal. Turn the growling into an opportunity to observe how wild the mind is.

Along with hunger pangs, you will most likely experience mood swings, low energy, and irritability during the first day or so of fasting. Most of the discomfort comes from the fact that your body is detoxifying at a rapid rate. During the first 36 hours of a fast, you will burn through all the glycogen stored in your liver. Then you will begin burning glycogen from your muscles, until your body goes into ketosis and switches over to burning fats. You can tell when you've switched to burning fats because your hunger pangs will go away and you will feel your brain fog clear and amazing lucidity take its place.

Fasting for three days is perfectly safe for most people in good health. If you have any concerns, check with your physician or health counselor before starting the vision quest. If you are diabetic, or taking medication, or dealing with acute illness, *do not* fast without first consulting a physician.

During your vision quest, listen to your body and follow its guidance. If at any time you feel sick, or your blood sugar is dropping dangerously, break your fast. I always keep chocolate and some basic foods like nuts and dried fruit in my vehicle, in case of emergency. Knowing there's chocolate just a few yards away makes it harder to maintain your fast, but you can turn this longing into a meditation—another opportunity to observe the madness of the mind.

Water: It's imperative to stay hydrated. You should drink at least four liters (about a gallon) of water a day, so plan accordingly when you pack your provisions. If you are making your vision quest in an arid desert climate, you will need more water—closer to six liters (a gallon and a half) a day.

The rule is to pee every hour. If you're not peeing that often, you're not drinking enough water.

Boredom: You will be bored. Take boredom as an indication that you are getting close to the state of contemplation you want to be in. Boredom and restlessness are the result of the limbic brain thrashing about for attention. Stay with the boredom, knowing that this is part of the process. Like hunger, it will pass.

Time: Leave your watch at home. Checking the time will not make it go by any faster, and you are trying to step into timelessness. Set your inner clock by the sun and the stars.

Meditation: During the day, you can do the exercise "I Am My Breath" in Chapter 12. In the evening, if you light a fire or a candle, you can do the exercise on burning old roles and identities described in Chapter 10. (If you do light a fire or candle, be sure there is no brush nearby that could ignite. And be sure the fire is extinguished completely and doused before you leave the area.)

Prayer: During your vision quest, pray, giving thanks for the beauty around you and for every breath you take. Give thanks for your hunger pangs or the wolves you are sure will devour you during the night. Practice praying with your heart and not with your head.

Ending your vision quest: Plan to end your three-day vision quest before nightfall on the third day. Before you leave the site, be sure to pick up all trash and carry it out with you. Make sure you leave the place as you found it—or cleaner. Leave no trace.

Breaking your fast: It's best to break your fast in the evening with a light vegetable broth or a miso soup, and then return to your regular gluten-free, dairy-free diet the following morning.

PART V

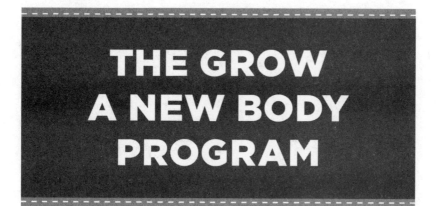

**THE GROW
A NEW BODY
PROGRAM**

Chapter 15

PREPARING FOR THE PROGRAM

Are you tired of feeling tired?
Have you had it with the brain fog and forgetfulness?
Tired of struggling with your weight?
Ready to reclaim your health?

Note: Do not do this program if you are pregnant or nursing, if you have cancer or a heart condition or any bowel disease. Consult with your doctor before starting this program.

The Grow a New Body Program Premises:

- You will heal your body with food.

- You will upgrade your brain with neuronutrients.

- You will know that what you eat and what you think determines how you feel, how you will grow old, and how you will die.

The Grow a New Body program is founded on a plant-based diet that's nutrient dense and calorie poor, low in protein and high in fats, and supported by superfoods and brain nutrients. For seven days only, you will offer your body supplements that switch on the longevity genes and detoxify the brain. And you will be on your way to growing a new body that ages slowly and gracefully, remains healthy, and avoids the heart disease, dementia, and cancers of modern civilization.

The program requires that you shed your stories the way the serpent sheds her skin; that you learn the jaguar-journey beyond death and honor the sacred feminine; that you find inner peace and stillness, and like the hummingbird feed only on the nectar of life; and that you discover an exalted personal vision and mission. Then, as you reach old age with a clear mind and a calm sense of a life well lived, you will step fearlessly into the beyond.

You do this by marrying cutting-edge neuroscience and biology with the ancient wisdom of the shamans.

Shamans and modern neuroscientists understand that we create our destiny (and our health or disease) by the unconscious beliefs stored in our LEF and in the neural networks in our brain. For example, beliefs like "the women in my mother's side die young" or "dementia runs in my family" become self-fulfilling prophecies. We can also change the beliefs that a "50 percent chance of developing Alzheimer's at the age of 85 is normal," or that "cancer and cardiovascular disease are natural." But upgrading these beliefs requires that we first upgrade our brains.

Years ago I asked an elderly medicine man in the Amazon rain forest what he did to avoid the diseases of old age. "Simple," he replied. "Live a long and healthy life." I laughed and said he had not understood the question: I wanted to know how to avoid the diseases of old age. He smiled and repeated the same answer.

Today I understand what he meant. The nutritional and spiritual practices that are an everyday ingredient of the shamanic way all support a belief in a long *and* healthy life. May this become your self-fulfilling prophecy!

The keys for unlocking the codes in your DNA for growing a new body are in the superfoods you will be taking—the Nrf2 activators. For these to work you first need to detox your brain, eliminating the environmental poisons you have ingested in your food, water, and air over the years.

The immediate benefits you can expect:

- Chronic health problems improve
- Many allergies improve or disappear
- Runny noses and headaches go away
- Blood sugar stabilizes
- You sleep better
- Joint pain and brain fog clears

By day three or four of the Grow a New Body program, many persons report dramatic decreases in their symptoms, from anxiety and depression, to joint pain to allergy relief. In many, 70 to 75 percent of their symptoms disappear by the end of the seven-day program. While I cannot guarantee you will experience these dramatic results, it is very likely that you will notice a significant difference in how you feel. You will be able to track your progress with the health questionnaire in Chapter 16. This questionnaire has been adapted from one developed by Dr. Mark Hyman that we use in our detox program (used with permission).

By the end of the week, you will have restarted your natural detoxification systems, the brain fog will disappear, and you will begin sleeping better. You will be on your way to growing a new body that ages and heals and dies differently.

After the program you will find that you can more easily dance between the visible, physical world of the senses and everyday tasks, and the invisible world of Spirit. You will be like the graceful jaguar, the balancing force of the rain forest who serves as an intermediary between the seen and unseen worlds.

How to Prepare for the Grow a New Body Program

If you are a consummate meat eater and are attached to your morning croissant and pasta dinners, you will need to change your eating habits to a primarily plant-based diet before you start the program. You will also need to go off sugar, dairy, and gluten.

Breaking the sugar habit is the most difficult. You will learn how to make your own potent probiotic to clear your system from the yeast menace *Candida albicans*. And you will repair your gut with probiotics and recover your "gut instincts." This will dramatically reduce your sugar cravings.

It's not only what you eat but when you eat that is important. You will reap the benefits of the daily 18-hour fast from sugars, and learn to use the powerful plant-based supplements that switch on the longevity genes and silence the genes that create disease.

You will discover how your high-protein diet may be leading you to an early death, and how to switch to a protein-restricted, primarily plant-based diet to ensure longevity and health.

After you have completed three weeks of preparation with the diet and supplements described in Chapter 6, you can begin the seven-day Grow a New Body program. The preparation will turn up the heat of your fat-burning engines and switch on the cascade of genes that create health and repair the body. Your system will be in mild ketosis. Once you start the Grow a New Body program, you will go into deep ketosis and regeneration.

Step 1. For three weeks, implement the diet and the supplements described in Chapter 6 and summarized in the next several pages, to begin to clear your body and brain from toxins, and turn on your fat-burning engines. Be sure you have eliminated sugars and anything that turns into sugar (simple carbohydrates) from your diet, as well as dairy and gluten. Do not attempt the Grow a New Body program without this preparation, as you can become toxic and feel quite ill.

Step 2. Start the Grow a New Body program. Your diet will consist of meals with very low protein, few carbs, and lots of healthy fats, a way of eating that will give your body an opportunity to switch on the longevity genes and the production of stem cells in your brain and other organs. Don't take any of your regular vitamins or supplements during the seven-day Grow a New Body program, but do take the powerful upregulators listed in this chapter. Continue taking any medication you are on.

After you complete the Grow a New Body program, return to the diet and supplements in Chapter 6. This diet will help you prevent the illnesses of the West, including dementia, heart disease, and cancer.

Step 3. Now you are ready to do your three-day vision quest, with only water to drink.

You can repeat the above steps every three months with the change of seasons. You can follow this plan for the rest of your long and healthy life:

Everyday Eating and Supplements When Not on the Grow a New Body Program

The Principles

- Practice the 18-hour daily fast from sugars or anything that turns into sugar in your gut, avoiding food from 6 P.M. to 12 P.M. the next day.
- Eat a primarily plant-based diet that's nutrient dense and calorie poor.
- Eat when you are hungry—small, frequent meals with good fats (omega-3 fats, olive oil, nuts, avocados).
- Avoid sugar and anything that turns into sugar (simple carbs) in your system.

- Reduce your protein intake to under 1 ounce (28 grams) per day, plant based, no animal protein or dairy. You want to downregulate mTOR as much as possible.

What to Do

- Drink 8 to 10 glasses of filtered water a day.
- Aim to have a bowel movement once or twice a day. Supplement with 2 tablespoons of flax seeds, probiotics, or up to 1,000 mg magnesium citrate, if needed.
- Sweat profusely at least three times during the week, using a sauna or steam room.
- Eat for color. Choose a rainbow assortment of vegetables rich in phytonutrients.
- Choose organic foods when possible.
- Eliminate meat and other animal foods.

What to Include

- Raw vegetables*; salads with avocados, olives
- Nuts (almonds, macadamia nuts, walnuts, hazelnuts, etc., but no peanuts)
- Nut butters (almond, cashew)
- Healthy oils (coconut, olive oil, cold-pressed nut oils)
- Spices and herbs, include ginger, turmeric, cilantro
- Onions and garlic
- Herbal teas (non-caffeinated)

If you'll be eating out, order grilled or steamed vegetables.

What to Avoid

- Dairy (milk, cheese, yogurt, butter, ghee)
- Red meat
- Gluten (barley, rye, oats, spelt, wheat, and other foods that contain gluten)

- Corn, soy, peanuts
- Vegetables in the deadly nightshade family (tomatoes, eggplants, peppers, potatoes)
- Sugars (table sugar, honey, maple syrup, corn syrup)
- Products containing or made with yeast (wine, vinegar, breads)

Everyday Supplements before the Grow a New Body Program

DHA: The dosage is 3 grams a day.
ALA: The dosage is 300 to 600 mg a day every three days.
Turmeric: The dosage is one gram a day in a liposomal form (or in foods like curries).
Vitamin B12: The dosage is 2,500 mcg a day.
Vitamin C: The dosage is one gram (1,000 mg) a day.
Vitamin D3: The dosage is 5,000 IU a day.
Coconut oil & MCT oil: The dosage is 2 tablespoons of each every morning and afternoon.
Ubiquinol: The dosage is 200 mg a day.
Multivitamin: Take the dosage indicated in the product.
Zinc: The dosage is 15 mg daily.
Magnesium: The dosage is 350 mg daily.
Calcium citrate: The dosage is 1,000 mg daily, on an empty stomach.
Vitamin K2: The dosage is 100 mcg daily.
Sodium bicarbonate: The dosage is ½ teaspoon in the evening two hours after your meal.
Nicotinamide riboside: The dosage is 100 mg daily.

Nutritional supplements are powerful substances and should be used with caution. If you choose to take the supplements above, consult with a physician or nutritionist. Be sure, when choosing supplements, that you favor gelcaps over capsules and capsules over tablets, to make it easier for your gut to absorb the ingredients.

The Seven-Day Grow a New Body Program Protocol

Without your knowledge or consent, you have been enrolled in the largest biology experiment in human history. It's the sugar-rich, nutrient-poor, highly acidic, processed-grain, GMO, meat-rich diet of Western countries. And the results of this experiment are becoming clear: Autism rates in the USA are now 1 in 12 boys,[1] 1 of 2 adults over the age of 85 will have diagnosable dementia,[2] 1 in 4 people will die of heart disease, and your chances for being diagnosed with cancer are nearly 40 percent.

You do not want to be part of this biology experiment. So you must conduct your own, with a sample size of one: You.

The guidelines that follow are the foundation of your experiment in exceptional health. It is not a one-size-fits-all solution, but rather a protocol that you must adjust to your individual biology. Be sure to listen to your body, adapt dosages to best suit your needs, and do your own research to find the best solutions for yourself.

The Menu: Eat Organic

The menu for the Grow a New Body program features fresh, fibrous vegetables; healthy nuts, seeds, and oils; and good fats like coconut and olive oil and avocados. These foods will provide plenty of the right kind of fats to fuel the brain. To support your gut-brain and your mitochondrial function (the power centers in your cells), try to get most of your fats from nuts, seeds, avocados, and healthy oils like coconut oil, cold-pressed extra-virgin olive oil, and flaxseed oil.

A home vacuum sealer will keep your food fresh for days in your refrigerator, and for months if frozen. It's a relatively inexpensive kitchen tool you'll wonder how you have managed to live without. I also like to keep Himalayan salt, pepper, extra-virgin olive oil, and vinegar at my office, so I can add these to my vegetables when I am ready to eat.

Be sure to have plenty of fibrous cruciferous vegetables like cauliflower, broccoli, Brussels sprouts, and cabbage. The cruciferous vegetables switch on the Nrf2 pathway and produce antioxidants and detox enzymes that turn on the longevity genes inside the cells. Avoid root vegetables, which have a high glycemic index, raising blood sugar levels.

Limit your fruit intake to small portions of frozen berries during the Grow a New Body program. Please follow the program below, and above all follow the wisdom of your body. If you find yourself getting achy, dizzy, or nauseous or developing headaches, stop the program, hydrate, and wait another week or two for your body to be better prepared.

Sample Meal Plan for the Grow a New Body Program

On waking	12 oz. glass of water with lemon, Green tea if desired, and *S. boulardii*
8 a.m.	Green juice
10 a.m.	Vegetable broth
11 a.m.	Smoothie (optional)
1 p.m.	Salad bar lunch
3 p.m.	Midafternoon snack (optional): nuts, seeds
6 p.m.	Dinner: a light, fiber-rich meal

On waking: Drink a 12-ounce glass of pure water, with half a lemon squeezed into it. This will help to set your body's pH, or body acidity/alkaline balance, to be a little more alkaline. An alkaline gut is a perfect environment for your gut flora to thrive and an uncomfortable environment for bad bugs and viruses. The typical Western diet is overabundant in acid-producing foods, resulting among other things in loss of bone density.

You can have green tea or a black tea, and you can use homemade almond milk in it if you like. You will find the recipe for almond milk in Chapter 17.

Next, have one tablespoon of homemade *S. boulardii* to compete with the Candida in your gut and reduce its population. This will keep you from getting *hangry* (hungry and irritable) during the seven-day Grow a New Body program.

When you find yourself getting hangry, it's the not-so-nice yeasts that are craving food (sugars) and releasing chemical compounds to trigger the hunger centers in the brain so that they can feed. Be sure to take the *S. boulardii* on an empty stomach. Otherwise, it will be feasting on the sugars in your gut and not doing the important work of displacing the Candida. Remember, you want this probiotic to nudge your Candida to move along through your GI tract to be excreted through your bowel movements.

8 A.M. Green juice. Green juice will provide phytochemicals in vegetables and fruits that have been shown to have cancer-preventive effects. They are pure natural wisdom, turning on the genes that create health and silencing the genes that create disease.

10 A.M. Vegetable broth. This broth is rich in the micronutrients that your body needs to repair. Include one tablespoon of MCT oil and coconut oil for ready fuel and to maintain nutritional ketosis.

11 A.M. Smoothie (optional). Your morning smoothie is rich in phytonutrients and good fats.

1 P.M. Salad lunch. When you buy organic produce for your salad, rinse the leafy greens and veggies and remember that their stalks and leaves are rich in earth-based probiotics. I don't use any commercial vegetable rinses. You can choose seeds and nuts to sprinkle on your salad.[3] Remember vegetable proteins! Broccoli has more protein per calorie than beef! During this program you want to avoid eggs. And keep your protein intake under 1 ounce (28 grams) per day. Fifty almonds contain about 1/2 ounce (14 grams) of good protein and lots of good fats!

3 P.M. Midafternoon snack (optional). Help yourself to olive tapenade on a celery stalk or a handful of nuts or seeds if you feel hunger pangs.

6 P.M. Dinner. A light, fiber-rich meal to feed your flora. Your dinner should be warm to make it easier to digest. Make sure it includes healthy fats: perhaps a spoonful of hummus (that contains nearly 1/4 ounce of protein) and olive tapenade with leafy greens sautéed in vegetable broth or coconut oil and a scoop of guacamole. I generally have a vegetable soup and salad for dinner, with lots of nuts and seeds, accompanied with avocado during the Grow a New Body program. Just be sure to finish all your eating for the day by 6 P.M. This will give you a full 18-hour period of fasting overnight, allowing your cells to go into autophagy, recycling useful amino acids.

To make dishes tastier, you can add nuts, seeds, and healthy oils, as well as fresh or dried herbs. Use flaxseed oil or extra-virgin olive oil only to flavor foods and dress salads, not for cooking, because they break down with heat. For cooking, use only coconut oil, which can withstand high temperatures.

Never boil vegetables or overcook them, as you'll break down the fiber and destroy the phytonutrients and vitamins. Instead, steam vegetables or sauté them in vegetable broth with herbs. Or coat them with coconut oil and grill them, without burning. Or eat them raw, drizzled with healthy oils.

Supplements for the Grow a New Body Program

During your seven-day Grow a New Body program, plan to take *only* the following supplements every day. Do not take any other vitamins or nutritional supplements during this time, unless directed by your health-care provider.

For more information on the supplements before and after your Grow a New Body program, see Chapter 6, Superfoods and Super Supplements.

It's very important that you take a break from your daily supplement regime during these seven days so your cells can focus their resources on detoxification, upgrade, and repair.

Morning

Trans-resveratrol: The dosage is 500 mg a day.

Pterostilbene: The dosage is 500 mg a day.

Curcumin, liposomal form: The dosage is 1,000 mg a day.

Sulforaphane: The dosage is 200 mg a day.

S-acetyl glutathione: The dosage is 1,000 mg a day.

Probiotic from ascended health: The dosage is 10 drops in water.

Coconut oil and MCT oil: Take a tablespoon of each with food in the morning and afternoon.

Vitamin B12: The dosage is 2,500 mcg a day.

Vitamin C: The dosage is 2,000 mg a day.

Zinc: The dosage is 30 mg a day.

Evening

Alpha-lipoic acid: The dosage is 600 mg a day.

Magnesium citrate: The dosage is 1,000 mg a day.

Herbal laxatives: As needed.

Morning Supplements to Take with Your Smoothie

Trans-resveratrol, a compound found in red wine, red grape skins, and certain berries, turns on longevity genes and triggers the production of antioxidants. Trans-resveratrol is the most bioavailable form of resveratrol, and boosts superoxide dismutase and glutathione, the brain's super antioxidants. The dosage is 500 mg a day.

Pterostilbene, found in blueberries and grapes, has been shown to lower cholesterol and glucose, and reduce blood pressure. Working together, pterostilbene and trans-resveratrol prevent cancer, heart disease, diabetes, and other illnesses. Trans-resveratrol works upstream, regulating the genes that activate apoptosis—programmed cell death, or cell suicide— while pterostilbene works downstream, turning off the genes that allow cancer cells to grow and proliferate. The dosage is 500 mg a day.

Curcumin, a phytochemical in the turmeric plant (a member of the ginger family), has extraordinary anti-inflammatory properties as well as regulating blood sugar, balancing cholesterol, and improving brain function. While you will be taking turmeric daily for its anti-inflammatory benefits, curcumin is much stronger and, to avoid overloading the body, should not be taken daily. Curcumin also switches on the SIRT-1 longevity genes and upregulates Nrf2. Take in liposomal form. In this case more is not better, and you do not want to take it for more than a week without giving it a rest for a few days. Remember that the Nrf2 pathway is dose dependent. The dosage is 1,000 mg a day in a liposomal form.

Sulforaphane is a naturally occurring organic sulfur that has anticancer properties and will help regenerate tissue, even bone. Sulforaphane is the star of the Nrf2 activators and detoxifiers, and three servings of broccoli per week will reduce the risk for prostate cancer by 60 percent![4] It is derived from glucoraphanin, when it comes into contact with the enzyme myrosinase, so be sure the supplement you purchase includes this enzyme. If it does not, take the sulforaphane with arugula, which is rich in this enzyme. Dr. Joe Mercola makes an excellent supplement you can purchase online that has myrosinase. I love to sprout broccoli seeds, because the three-day-old sprouts contain up to 100 times higher concentrations of glucoraphanin than the broccoli florets. Due to its low molecular weight, sulforaphane has the greatest bioavailability of all the Nrf2 activators. If you are serious about growing a new body, grow your own sprouts. It is easy and fun. The dosage is 200 mg daily.

S-acetyl glutathione is the first truly bioavailable form of glutathione, which scavenges free radicals. It protects DNA from damage and is crucial for energy metabolism and optimal mitochondrial function.[5] It also supports detoxification of the liver, lungs, kidneys, and other organs.[6] Dosage is 1,000 mg a day.

Probiotics resettle healthy flora in the gut and facilitate digestion. I use Active Detox Probiotic as they are extraordinary, but you can use another high-quality probiotic as well. Take 10 drops in water. You can order Active Detox Probiotic at www.ascendedhealth.com. Follow dosage on label.

Coconut oil and MCT oil are jet fuel for the brain. Take 1 tablespoon of each in the morning and in the midafternoon.

Vitamin B12 is essential for liver detoxification and for preserving intact DNA, important for cell growth. Most Americans are B12 deficient. Be sure to take sublingual methylcobalamin, an enhanced form of B12 that dissolves quickly under the tongue. The dosage is 2,500 micrograms (mcg) a day.

Vitamin C is essential for detoxification processes. The dosage is 2,000 mg a day.

Zinc is needed by the liver to detox. The World Health Organization estimates that one in three people is deficient in zinc. The dosage is 30 mg a day.

Evening (two hours after dinner):

Alpha-lipoic acid helps eliminate toxins and heavy metals embedded in brain tissue. The dosage is 600 mg a day.

Magnesium citrate helps with bowel movements and eliminating waste. It also relaxes your muscles. The dosage is 1,000 mg a day.

Herbal laxatives can help you keep a regular bowel movement as needed. Be sure that you are moving your bowels at least once a day.

What to Expect

For the first two or three days of your Grow a New Body program, it's normal to feel tired, achy, and uncomfortable or experience gas, bad breath, or headaches while you are eliminating toxins. Drinking plenty of water will help speed the process of flushing out toxins through your kidneys. You will also eliminate through the skin, so you can expect to sweat more than usual. For the first few days, allow yourself extra rest. You might want to schedule the start of your program around a weekend.

Don't be surprised if you experience brain fog and difficulty focusing during the first couple of days. Toxins are stored in the fat in the brain, and your brain will begin to release them into your bloodstream so you can eliminate them through your bowels.

You may also feel irritable and moody. Physical detox tends to loosen up long-buried emotions. I'm convinced that toxic emotions bind to physical toxins, and your body will be working hard at clearing out the physical and emotional poisons. Pay attention to any feelings or memories that surface during this time—you may reexperience old hurts. Try not to be reactive: This is not the time to make big decisions or confront others about personal issues. Instead, take time to honor emotions that are being released. Often, they will resolve by themselves as the body detoxifies.

I recommend journaling about your thoughts and feelings, so that the people around you don't have to bear the brunt of any irritability you may feel. Journaling will also help you gain perspective on past sorrows that may surface, help release old hurts, and may bring you to a feeling of forgiveness. In fact, in a few days, as your head starts to clear, you're likely to have a very different take on old problems.

After day four you will begin to feel a dawning sense of clarity you have not felt in a long time as the brain fog clears (even if you did not think you had any brain fog before). You will notice your mood lifting and your digestion improving. The little aches (and some of the big ones as well) will start to go away, and your allergies, if you have any, will begin to improve.

Because your body is functioning better, you may find that you're sleeping less but feeling more rested.

Sometime between day four and day five, you will find that you have a surprisingly large bowel movement and wonder how this could be, given how little you are eating. This is because your body is eliminating toxins that have been stored inside cells and have made their way down into your GI tract. Be sure to keep your bowels moving daily!

Around day five you will notice that your perception of the world has changed. The colors will seem brighter, the air crisper, your mood lighter, and your life more beautiful. By day seven your higher brain will have become engaged and you will find that many of your questions answer themselves as they form inside your head. Your blood sugar will begin to stabilize at a healthy level, and your food cravings will be largely gone. You will have set in motion dormant programs in your DNA that will turn on the production of stem cells in every organ in your body.

Monitoring Your Progress

One way to monitor your progress is to track your fasting glucose levels. You can do this with a glucometer, which you can buy for about $10 at a drugstore.

Test your blood sugar in the morning before eating anything. An ideal glucose level should be between 75 and 90 mg/dl—ideally, below 85. Two hours after you drink your 11 A.M. smoothie and before you eat your noon meal, test your glucose level again. It should be no more than 40 points above what it was before you ate. While a fasting glucose of 105 is considered normal, to avoid diabetes and dementia, aim for a lower level. To trigger the SIRT-1 genes and grow a new body, an ideal glucose level is around 75 to 80 mg/dl.

To get an accurate reading of how your glucose levels change, test your blood sugar level daily for a few days before starting the Grow a New Body program, during the program, and afterward.

As you change your diet to fuel your brain on fats and nutrient-rich plants, test your blood sugar periodically. As you lower your glucose levels, you are extending your health span.

The Grow a New Body protocol will also lower your IGF-1 levels, reducing your chances of developing cancer and other diseases. When we do blood-chemistry tests on participants in our program, we find that their levels of IGF-1 drop between 30 and 50 percent in just seven days.

Research cardiologists at the Intermountain Medical Center Heart Institute found that fasting lowers the risk of coronary artery disease and diabetes, the leading cause of death in America. Even a 24-hour fast will increase the levels of human growth hormone, which repairs the body and maintains metabolic balance, by a staggering 1,300 percent in men and 2,000 percent in women.[7] And on the Grow a New Body program, you will be fasting daily from 6 P.M. to 12 noon the following day.

Be Patient

Remember that detoxifying and upgrading your body is a process. Your limbic brain—the tyrant king—will most likely rebel against your efforts to remove it from its sugar and dopamine-rich throne as the driver of your decisions, emotions, and perceptions. It may insist that nothing's happening, so why bother continuing the program? Whatever excuse your primitive brain proffers, don't give in to its insistent voice!

Above all, be patient with yourself during the program. Your gut can't repair itself without a little discomfort, and you can't reverse years of bad habits in a few days. But the payoff of even a small positive change is that you'll feel far better very quickly—generally within the first few days—and that will prime you to continue a healthier way of living. ·

Other Aids to Detoxification: Baths, Brushing, and Saunas

The skin is one of the main organs involved in detoxification. You can speed the process of eliminating toxins with detox baths, saunas, or skin brushing.

Detox baths work by stimulating the body to release toxins through the skin. You literally sweat them out. Very warm water will cause you to sweat, and Epsom salts, which isn't really a type of salt but magnesium sulfate, can be added to warm bathwater to help with the process. The magnesium is absorbed into your system and helps move toxins through your body and out your liver. Epsom salts promote healthy circulation and better utilization of oxygen and minerals—and can lower blood pressure and reduce inflammation. As an added bonus, Epsom salts will relax your muscles, easing stress.

Adding essential oils to your detox bath will relax you even more. Lavender oil has a scent that has been shown to release muscle tension. Other ingredients you might add to your bath, alone or in combination, are baking soda, apple cider vinegar, and Himalayan salt, all of which can aid in detoxing through the skin.

Remain in the detox bath for about 20 minutes. Be especially careful getting out of the tub so you don't fall because your relaxed muscles might not adjust quickly as you stand to exit the bath.

Saunas can also enhance the skin's ability to detoxify. A conventional sauna, which circulates hot air, causes breathing problems for some people and is not as effective at aiding detoxification as a far-infrared sauna. *Far* refers to the position at the extreme end of the light spectrum, and far-infrared rays that are used in this type of sauna actually penetrate your skin to a depth of about one inch, helping release toxins stored under the epidermis.

Skin brushing stimulates circulation, which helps with detoxification. Before or during your detox bath, brush the skin all over your body. You can buy a brush for this purpose at a health-food store or online. Just be sure to clean the brush regularly and allow it to dry fully between uses.

Shamanic Meditations

Our doctors tell us that we are the product of our genetics—if heart disease runs in your family, you have risk factors that predispose you to this condition. And our psychologists tell us that we are the product of our childhood and of our family dramas. This is true, these are the default programs that play out in our love stories and our health histories. But it does not *have* to be so.

In the instant of your conception, your genetic destiny was set. In the brief minutes when your father's sperm burrowed into your mother's egg, you received 23 chromosomes from your mother and 23 chromosomes from your father. You did not get to choose strong heart and good brains, nature selected for you. And as we know, sometimes these choices have left a lot to be desired.

During your vision quest in nature, you can go back and visit the moment of your conception, and have a say about the genes and qualities that you inherited. Of course we know that we cannot travel to the past, to the time before we were born. Yet the following exercise will help you select for the expression of your genes that bring you a good heart, strong bones, and healthy brain. In fact, you do not have to believe in time travel for this powerful visualization to work. You only have to be open to the experience, and know that visualization can not only improve athletic performance, it can improve your health. And just as important, you can forgive your parents for any transgressions you believe they committed toward you, and any hurt you feel they might have imposed on you.

This is crucial for growing a new body, because holding on to any residual anger or resentment toward your parents only keeps you as a victim of their genetic signatures.

You can record the journey (every phone today has this option) and then listen to your recording while in nature.

EXERCISE
SOUL RETRIEVAL IN NATURE DURING VISION QUEST

Soul retrieval helps us shed limiting beliefs, traumatic experiences, and the tired old stories from our childhood and upbringing. As you return to a more authentic self, you can better serve the biological process to grow a new body.

With your eyes closed, take a few deep, relaxing breaths. Count your breaths from one to ten, then back to one again, until you feel yourself entering a deep state of relaxation.

Now imagine your timeline, the chronology of the events of your life, in front of you like in a movie screen. Perhaps you see a golden thread or a string with many beads or moments of time. Perhaps you simply see a road that leads in one direction to the past and another direction forward into the future.

Imagine that you can travel along your timeline, briefly revisiting events of the past few days. Go further into the past, to the last few weeks and months, and then the last few years, all the way to your childhood, and to your earliest memories as a toddler. See the images as though they are in a movie that you can fast-forward or reverse at will.

When you are no longer able to recall events or situations, use your imagination. Imagine yourself as a baby in your mother's arms. Imagine being inside her womb. Imagine the instant of your conception, when your mother's egg is surrounded by your father's numerous sperm, all trying to fertilize it.

Imagine yourself sitting inside that luminous egg. It is a peaceful bubble. Know that you are filling it with your peace and luminosity. And now notice the blinding light that occurs at the moment of conception. Observe how the egg has invited the finest sperm to fertilize it. Imagine it entering into the ovum, and you witness the most extraordinary alchemy that is the conception of you.

The nuclei of the sperm and the egg dissolve into each other, and your father's DNA and your mother's DNA fuse. In the blink of an eye, the egg divides and forms two tiny, identical cells. They begin to replicate, doubling, quadrupling, and exponentially adding to their numbers at an extraordinary rate.

As you watch this amazing process, you hold steadfast to your intention calling forth the best qualities from your mother's line. The courage of your grandmothers, the strength of the women in your father's side. The grandfather that was perfectly clear-headed in his 90s. You bathe these nascent cells with your great peace, your serenity, your light. You fill this holy union that is you with love and forgiveness, regardless of what the "facts" of your conception may have been.

And there, then, you forgive your parents. You see them as holy, glorious, innocent beings. You bathe them with your love, knowing that all is well.

Now return along your timeline, visiting your childhood and pausing at any major traumatic event that you encounter. Observe that frightened you and reach out to him or her, letting them know that all will be okay, that they are loved and cared for. Notice how they recognize you, making eye contact with you as you reach back to them from the future to encourage them with your love. Continue making your way to the present, bringing with you—into the here and now—your feelings of peace and luminosity, your joy and exhilaration, your innocence and playfulness, your ability to trust and to play.

Welcome yourself back home.

Crafting a New Epic Life Story

We have two principal great stories that shape our destiny. One is written in our DNA code and predisposes us to live, get sick, and die the way that our parents did. The other is the story we tell ourselves and others about who we are, where we came from, and where we are headed.

The following exercise will show you how to become the author of a more creative and powerful story that defines your life journey.

Exercise
The Story of Your Life

In your journal write a one-page fairy tale that starts with "Once upon a time. . . ." Include at least these three characters: a princess or prince, a warrior, and a dragon. If you think this sounds childish, give yourself permission to be childlike for a few moments.

Read your story aloud to a friend or partner and look for themes. What genre is it: adventure, romance, a tale of despair, or a quest for love or fortune? Who is the main character: the princess, the dragon, or another character?

Now change the tense from past to present and claim all actions of every character. For example, you might change, "And then the prince left his father so he could journey across the sea to unknown lands," to "And then I left my father . . . ."

Notice how the tone and significance of the story changes. Like in a dream, where all the characters are a mirror for one aspect of ourselves, all the characters in this story are part of you. Observe the tests and challenges that you face and how you succeed or fail to overcome them.

Now rewrite the story, casting your character as a hero or heroine who embarks upon a journey in search of invisible treasures. For example, you, as the princess, change from someone who abandons her family when her father's castle is under siege to, instead, a maiden who follows her heart's calling to explore the world and discover her purpose in life, and the wisdom that will help her become queenly.

Then read your rewritten story as the parable it is. Identify with the lessons and gifts you experience in your story—and in your life.

Remember that we are our stories, and the tales that we believe about ourselves become flesh and bone. As you become the author of a new and more meaningful story, visualize your brain laying new pathways for lifelong health, joy, inner peace, and enlightenment.

Chapter 16

GROW A NEW BODY HEALTH QUESTIONNAIRE

This questionnaire has been adapted from one developed by Dr. Mark Hyman that we use in our detox programs (used with permission).

Please score the symptoms you have experienced in the last month. Score yourself before and after completing the Grow a New Body program.

Point Scale

0 = Never or almost never experience this

1 = Occasionally, not severe

2 = Occasionally, severe

3 = Frequently, not severe

4 = Frequently, severe

HEAD

_____Headaches   _____Dizziness

_____Faintness   *Total* _____

BRAIN

_____Poor memory   _____Slurred speech

_____Confusion   _____Forgetfulness

_____Poor concentration   _____Learning disability

_____Poor coordination   *Total* _____

MOUTH/THROAT

_____Chronic coughing   _____Soreness, loss of voice

_____Constantly clearing   _____Swollen tongue, gums
throat

_____Canker sores   *Total* _____

EYES

_____Watery, itchy eyes   _____Bags, dark circles

_____Swollen, reddened eyes *Total* _____

NOSE

_____Stuffy nose   _____Sneezing attacks

_____Sinus congestion   _____Excessive mucus

_____Hay fever   _____Frequent colds

Total _____

EARS

_____Itchy ears   _____Drainage from ears

_____Earaches, ear infections _____Ringing, hearing loss

Total _____

DIGESTIVE

_____Nausea or vomiting   _____Bloated feeling

_____Reflux   _____Belching or passing gas

_____Diarrhea   _____Heartburn

_____Constipation   _____Intestinal/stomach pain

Total _____

LUNGS

_____Chest congestion   _____Shortness of breath

_____Asthma, bronchitis   _____Difficulty breathing

Total _____

SKIN

_____Acne   _____Flushing, hot flashes

_____Hives, rash, dry skin   _____Excessive sweating

_____Hair loss   _Total_ _____

JOINTS/MUSCLES

_____Pain or aches   _____Limitation of movement

_____Arthritis   _____Weakness or tiredness

_____Stiffness   _____Fatigue

                               Total _____

WEIGHT

_____Binge eating/drinking   _____Compulsive eating

_____Craving sweets   _____Water retention

_____General food cravings   _____No appetite

                               Total _____

EMOTIONS

_____Mood swings   _____Depression

_____Anxiety, fear, nervous _____Difficulty deciding

_____Anger, irritability   _____Obsessive thoughts

                               Total _____

HEART

_____Irregular heartbeat _____Chest pain

_____Rapid or pounding _____High blood pressure

Total _____

SLEEP

_____Insomnia _____Tossing and turning

_____Hard to get to sleep _____Nightmares

_____Wake up in the night _____Hard to wake up

Total _____

ENERGY/ACTIVITY

_____Fatigue/sluggishness _____Hyperactivity

_____Apathy, lethargy _____Restlessness

Total _____

Grand Total _____

Add individual scores and total each group. Add group scores to give a grand total.

Optimal is less than 10

Mild toxicity 10–50

Moderate toxicity 50–100

Severe toxicity over 100

Chapter 17

RECIPES FOR INNER HEALING

The world does not need another recipe book. There are dozens of ways to prepare a smoothie, and you already probably have found one that you like best. The recipes in this chapter are the ones mentioned in the book, and are basic ideas that you can improve on. Add the ingredients that will make them distinctly yours, and that make you happy.

These recipes were developed at the Center for Energy Medicine in Chile, where we have world-class chefs preparing meals, and they turn out exquisitely. But remember that the Grow a New Body program is not an invitation to a banquet. It is designed to stress your system in subtle ways so that it will respond creatively by going into repair and regeneration mode.

This is not dinner at your favorite Italian restaurant. The program is mimicking a starvation diet, yet with ample nutrients available to your system.

HOMEMADE *S. BOULARDII*

It is simple to grow your own strain of the probiotic *Saccharomyces boulardii (S. boulardii)*, which can help you dramatically reduce your gut's population of *Candida albicans*. The *S. boulardii* are living organisms, and they will respond to your thoughts and feelings. I like to say a blessing over them in the same way that I say a prayer over my food before a meal.

After you prepare a batch, you can use a spoonful of your *S. boulardii* as a starter for the next batch. Here's what you need to do:

- Gather about 4 cups of organic, ripe fruit from your garden or grocer. The overripe fruit your market is going to pull from the case is best, as it is loaded with sugars. I love using blueberries or raspberries, but they must be very ripe. Pears, mangoes, and frozen berries work great. If needed, pit the fruit (e.g., apples), but do not peel it.

- Blend the fruit in a blender with 1 cup of spring water.

- Cook the fruit and water mixture in a saucepan at low heat until it boils for 20 minutes.

- Let the batch cool to body temperature. Then, add the contents of 2 gelatin capsules of *S. boulardii*. Get the best-quality brand you can find. I like Klaire Labs and Pure Encapsulations.

- Pour the mixture into a large bowl, filling it halfway. The batch will expand as it ferments, so you want to be sure it has plenty of room to grow.

- Place the bowl in your oven, but don't turn the oven on. The heat from the oven light is all you will need to keep the mixture at body temperature for the next two or three days.

- Watch as your batch of *S. boulardii* grows and ferments, making strong medicine for you!

After two to three days, the *S. boulardii* will have fermented all the sugars in the fruit. You might want to taste it on day two. When there is no residue of sweet taste, you know it is ready. Place the mixture in the refrigerator and use one tablespoon daily before breakfast for two weeks before the Grow a New Body program, and as needed thereafter. Your *S. boulardii* will last for two weeks in the refrigerator, as the minute amounts of alcohol in the batch will preserve it.

BREAKFAST

Green Goddess Juice

2 Servings

I use an Omega Juicer to make this extraordinary juice every morning, as a blender will turn it into a smoothie. I am interested in the phytonutrients, not the fiber, which I will have with the smoothie a couple of hours later.

In this delicious drink, the spinach is mild, the kale is tangy, the lemon and ginger add a bite, and the cucumber is full of minerals.

1 cup baby spinach leaves

1 cup kale leaves

¼ green apple, with core removed

1 small handful parsley leaves and stems

1 medium cucumber

½-inch piece fresh ginger

½ medium lemon

Chop all ingredients so they go into the juicer easily. Cut the peel off the lemon, leaving the white flesh. Cut lemon into quarters. Juice all ingredients, adding lemon last, to suit your taste. If you are new to the taste of ginger, add a small portion and increase gradually.

Green Smoothie

2 Servings

½ cup spinach

½ cup kale

1 cucumber, peeled

½ or 1 lemon, peeled and chopped, to taste

1-inch piece fresh ginger

1 handful mint leaves

1/2 green apple, cored

2 cups filtered water

1 tablespoon MCT oil

1 tablespoon coconut oil

1 small ripe avocado, without pit or skin

Blend the spinach, kale, cucumber, lemon, ginger, mint, apple, and water in a blender. Add the avocado and oils at the end, and then stir. This is a very potent mix. If it is too strong, add a bit more cucumber.

Variation: You can replace the water with a cup of homemade almond milk. You can make almond milk by adding about 12 raw almonds that have soaked in water overnight to one cup of water and then mixing in a blender until smooth.

Morning Broth

6 Servings

2 sliced carrots

1 large chopped onion

1 cup daikon root and tops

1 cup winter squash cut in cubes

1 cup turnips

2 cups chopped greens (include kale, beet greens, or chard)

4 celery stalks

1 cup seaweed

1 cup cabbage

Sea salt to taste

1 cup fresh or dried shiitake mushrooms

Boil 2 quarts of water in a large soup pot. Add all the ingredients. Cover and bring to a gentle boil for 20 minutes. Lower the heat and simmer for 1 hour. Strain and enjoy.

After cooling, the broth can be stored in glass containers and refrigerated for consumption throughout the week.

LUNCH

During the seven-day Grow a New Body program, you will undoubtedly have lunch appointments. When you go out for lunch, above all do not eat the bread. Order salad and fresh seasonal vegetables, grilled. If you need to eat out, make an effort to choose a restaurant that is known for its fresh, organic, local ingredients so you can easily stay on your program.

Home Salad Bar

The lunch salad bar is fantastic if you take the time to prepare and to shop carefully. I like to store my salad-bar ingredients in glass jars on my counter top (the ones that need no refrigeration) and in resealable baggies in the fridge for the ones that need to be kept cool.

You can cut veggies into bite-size pieces and select the day's salad in the morning before going to work. Select different options each day, and vacuum seal your lunch. Refrigerate at work until ready to eat.

Be sure to use greens as your base, adding veggies and fats (and proteins) on top.

VEGETABLES	
Artichoke hearts	Scallions
Broccoli	Snap peas
Cucumbers	Sprouts (You can make your own bean sprouts at home.)
Herbs—oregano, cilantro, basil, and dill to taste	Steamed asparagus
Mushrooms (cooked)	Sun-dried tomatoes
Radishes	Zucchini

GREENS	
Arugula	Mixed baby greens
Kale	Spinach

FATS AND PROTEIN	
Avocado or guacamole (as much as you want)	Olive tapenade
Hummus	Seeds—pumpkin, sunflower, chia, hemp, sesame, etc.
Nuts—cashews, almonds, walnuts, etc.	Walnut tapenade

DRESSINGS AND DIPS	
Guacamole	Salad Dressing
Kale	Spinach

DRESSINGS AND DIPS

Salad Dressing

6 Servings

½ cup extra-virgin olive oil

¼ cup lemon juice

2 tablespoons chopped fresh herbs (such as parsley, tarragon, chives, basil, cilantro, and oregano)

1 teaspoon Dijon mustard

Blend all ingredients in a small food processor or whisk together.

Guacamole

4 to 6 Servings

2 ripe Hass avocados

½ teaspoon Himalayan salt or sea salt

3 tablespoons fresh lemon juice

¼ cup minced red onion

2 tablespoons cilantro (leaves), finely chopped

Dash of freshly ground black pepper

2 garlic cloves, finely chopped

Dash of paprika

1 sun-dried tomato soaked in water (or more, to taste)

Cut the avocados in half, and remove the pits. Scoop out the flesh with a spoon. Using a fork, mash the avocados. Sprinkle with salt and lemon juice.

Soak the minced red onion in cold water with a dash of salt for 10 minutes, then drain. This will lessen the intensity of the onions.

Add the minced onion, cilantro, black pepper, garlic, and paprika to the mashed avocados.

Chop the sun-dried tomato and add to your guacamole just before serving.

Hummus

4 Servings

2 cups chickpeas

3 garlic cloves

⅓ cup tahini

4 to 8 drops of hot sauce

1 large lemon, juice only

2 to 4 tablespoons filtered water

1 teaspoon Himalayan salt or sea salt

2 tablespoon extra-virgin olive oil

¼ teaspoon paprika

If using canned chickpeas, rinse then drain. (If using raw chickpeas, see instructions below.) Warm chickpeas in a pot over medium heat until heated thoroughly. Transfer to a blender or food processor. Add garlic, tahini, hot sauce, lemon juice, and 2 tablespoons water. Blend until the hummus is pureed, adding more water as needed.

Add Himalayan salt to taste. Place in a serving bowl and top with olive oil and paprika.

You can keep the hummus in a sealed container in the refrigerator for 5 days.

To cook raw chickpeas: Soak chickpeas in enough water to cover for 4 hours and rinse. Place 1/4 onion, one clove of garlic, a dash of paprika, a dash of curcumin powder, a dash of black pepper, and a sprig of celery in a pot, and then cover in cold water. Cook at medium heat until the chickpeas are soft. When the mixture boils, skim off and discard the foam with a spoon.

Olive Tapenade

6 Servings

I like to use kalamata olives for this delicious tapenade, but this is a good opportunity to taste the different olives in your market's olive bar. Be sure that they are brine-cured.

1½ cups pitted olives

¼ cup capers

2 teaspoons chopped parsley

2 cloves roasted garlic

Juice from 2 lemons

½ teaspoon black pepper

1 teaspoon anchovy paste (optional)

¼ cup extra-virgin olive oil

Himalayan salt to taste

Place olives, capers, parsley, garlic, lemon juice, black pepper, and anchovy paste, if using, in a food processor. Blend until coarsely chopped.

Add olive oil and blend until a coarse paste develops. Be sure to leave olive chunks; do not overblend. Add salt to taste.

Walnut Tapenade

6 Servings

¼ cup sun-dried tomatoes

1 cup walnuts, toasted in the oven for 10 minutes at 360°F

¼ cup fresh parsley

2 cloves garlic

¼ teaspoon salt

¼ teaspoon ground black pepper

½ cup extra-virgin olive oil

½ cup kalamata olives (optional)

Place sun-dried tomatoes in boiling water for 10 minutes, and then drain.

Place all ingredients in a blender, and blend until well mixed but maintain a chunky consistency.

Taste and season with salt and pepper as needed.

The tapenade will last for 1 week when refrigerated.

SOUPS

Roasted Butternut Squash Soup

6 Servings

This soup is rich in potassium, helping to prevent bone loss. And it is delicious.

1 large butternut squash halved (top to bottom) and seeded

2 tablespoons coconut oil

¾ teaspoon salt

¾ teaspoon freshly ground black pepper, or to taste

½ cup chopped shallots

4 garlic cloves, minced

¼ teaspoon ground nutmeg

3 cups organic vegetable broth

2 tablespoons extra-virgin olive oil

Preheat oven to 425°F. Place the butternut squash on a pan. Coat the inside of the squash with 1 tablespoon coconut oil. Sprinkle with ½ teaspoon salt and pepper.

Roast the squash facedown until it is tender, about 45 minutes.

Place on a cutting board and let the squash cool for 10 minutes, then scoop flesh into a bowl and discard the skin.

Warm remaining 1 tablespoon coconut oil in a skillet over medium heat and add the chopped shallots and 1/4 teaspoon salt. Cook 4 minutes, stirring, until the shallots turn golden, then add the garlic and cook about 1 minute, stirring.

Place the cooked garlic and shallots in a high-speed blender. Carefully add the squash flesh, nutmeg, and 1/4 teaspoon black pepper, and blend with vegetable broth until creamy.

Place soup in saucepan and cook at medium heat for 10 minutes. Top each serving with a sprinkling of olive oil and black pepper.

Los Lobos Vegetable Soup

6 Servings

This is our basic hardy everyday recipe, and in winter I will add a touch of smoked paprika. A good soup gets better the day after you prepare it, and will last 2 or 3 days in the refrigerator. You want to use ingredients that are fresh and seasonal.

1 tablespoon coconut oil

2 cups chopped onions

8 cloves garlic, minced

1 large carrot, diced

¼ teaspoon freshly ground black pepper

2 bay leaves

6 cups filtered water

1 large stalk celery, minced

1 cup chopped cabbage

½ pound fresh mushrooms, sliced

2 teaspoons salt

1½ cups tomato juice or 3/4 cup tomato sauce

1 medium ripe tomato, diced

6 scallions, minced

1 medium zucchini, diced

1 handful spinach

Pinch of dried basil, dill, and thyme

Place coconut oil in a large soup pot and add onion, garlic, carrot, pepper, and 1 bay leaf and saute for 30 seconds at medium heat. Add 6 cups of water, cover, and bring to a boil for 20 minutes at medium heat, and add remaining ingredients. Simmer for one hour. Cool and serve.

Rich Avocado Soup

6 Servings

This cold soup is one of my favorites for warm days, and it's rich in good fats. The benefit of a raw soup like this one is that none of the enzymes or vitamins has been compromised, as there is no heat in the preparation.

4 cucumbers, peeled, seeded, and chopped

3 ripe Hass avocados, peeled

½ cup fresh cilantro, chopped

¼ cup fresh lemon juice

½ teaspoon smoked paprika

½ cup filtered water

¼ teaspoon salt

½ red bell pepper, cut into strips for garnish

Place the cucumbers, avocados, cilantro, lemon juice, paprika, water, and salt into a high-speed blender and process until you reach a smooth consistency. Season to taste. Place in the refrigerator for at least one hour before serving. Ladle the soup into bowls and garnish each with a strip of bell pepper.

SIDE DISHES AND DINNER

Here are the ingredients and recipes for the dinner plan. Make dinner an occasion, even if you are eating by yourself. Remember that you are nourishing your body and feeding your soul. Light a candle, set the table nicely, and remember that a feast is about quality, not quantity!

Brussels Sprouts Stir-Fry

6 Servings

I have to admit I used to not like Brussels sprouts—that is, until I tried a variation of this recipe at True Food Kitchen in Los Angeles. The secret is to use small, fresh, young sprouts and to not

252

overcook them. Brussels sprouts are loaded with Nrf2 activators and rich in anti-inflammatory phytonutrients.

1 ½ teaspoons coconut oil

1 ½ pounds small Brussels sprouts, sliced in halves

3 garlic cloves, sliced thin

¼ cup filtered water

2 teaspoons fresh-squeezed

lemon juice

½ teaspoon fresh grated lemon zest

¼ teaspoon Himalayan salt

¼ teaspoon freshly ground black pepper

Heat a skillet over high heat and add the coconut oil until it is completely melted. Add the Brussels sprouts and garlic. Sauté for 1 minute until browned. Add water carefully, and cook for 2 minutes with a cover, after stirring the sprouts in the pan. Remove the cover and stir in the lemon juice, lemon zest, salt, and pepper. Continue to cook for another 7 or 8 minutes until tender. Serve hot.

Zucchini Pasta

2 Servings

2 zucchini, peeled

1 tablespoon coconut oil

2 garlic cloves, sliced

¼ cup filtered water

¼ teaspoon Himalayan salt

Freshly ground black pepper to taste

Olive oil, as garnish

Cut zucchini into thin slices using a vegetable peeler, stopping when you reach the seeds. (You can also use a mandoline for this task.)

Heat coconut oil in a skillet over medium heat; add in zucchini and garlic and stir for 1 minute. Add water in small amounts, adding more and continuing to cook until zucchini is soft and all the water is evaporated, 5 to 7 minutes.

Season with salt and pepper, and sprinkle olive oil on top. Add your favorite pesto or tapenade if you like. Serve hot.

Grilled Asparagus

2 Servings

1 pound fresh asparagus

2 tablespoons coconut oil

¼ teaspoon salt

¼ teaspoon freshly ground pepper

2 tablespoons extra-virgin olive oil

Preheat the oven to 425°F. Place the asparagus in an oven pan, and drizzle with the coconut oil. Toss to coat the spears, then sprinkle with salt and pepper. Bake in the preheated oven until tender, about 12 to 15 minutes. Add olive oil liberally before serving.

Steamed Broccoli

2 Servings

1 bunch broccoli (about ¾ pound)

1 clove garlic, chopped

1½ tablespoons olive oil

1 ½ teaspoons fresh lemon juice

Salt, to taste

Pepper, to taste

Chop broccoli into 2-inch florets. Steam broccoli in a steamer, covered, for 4 to 5 minutes until tender.

While broccoli is cooking, combine garlic with olive oil, lemon juice, and salt and pepper in a small skillet. Cook on medium heat until garlic is fragrant, 2 to 3 minutes. Make sure that the olive oil does not begin to smoke. Toss broccoli with garlic mixture and serve.

Perfect Quinoa

6 Servings

1 cup quinoa

1 ½ cups filtered water

2 capsules *S. boulardii* (or 1 table-spoon of the homemade variety)

¼ teaspoon salt

1 tablespoon extra-virgin olive oil

Rinse the quinoa in a fine mesh colander under running cold water for at least 30 seconds, until all the foam rinses off. Place in a pan with warm water and add *S. boulardii*. Cover and leave overnight. The *S. boulardii* with neutralize anti-nutrients in the quinoa and turn it into a superfood.

Twenty-four hours later, bring the quinoa to a boil over medium-high heat, then lower to a simmer. Cook uncovered about 10 minutes until the quinoa has absorbed all the water. Remove from heat and cover pot, allowing the quinoa to steam for 5 minutes.

Fluff the quinoa with a fork. Add salt to taste. Serve with a drizzle of extra-virgin olive oil.

The quinoa will last 4 days in the refrigerator.

Vegetable Stir-Fry

2 Servings

1 tablespoon coconut oil

1 medium onion, sliced thin

½ red bell pepper, cut into strips

¼ cup diagonally sliced carrots

½ cup broccoli florets

¼ cup thinly sliced zucchini

¼ cup snap peas

1 teaspoon sesame oil

1 tablespoon soy sauce

4 garlic cloves, sliced

1-inch piece gingerroot, grated

Heat the coconut oil in a wok or deep skillet on medium high. Add onions, bell peppers, and carrots and stir-fry for 2 minutes. Add the remaining vegetables and stir-fry for 5 to 7 minutes or until tender.

Add the sesame oil, soy sauce, garlic, and ginger. Mix well and stir-fry for 2 minutes.

YOUR DINNER PLAN	
Day 1:	Los Lobos Vegetable Soup 1 tablespoon Walnut Tapenade 4 celery stalks for dipping the tapenade Grilled Asparagus
Day 2:	Rich Avocado Soup Brussels Sprout Stir-Fry 1 tablespoon Olive Tapenade 1 tablespoon Hummus 4 celery stalks for dipping the tapenade or hummus
Day 3:	Salad mixed greens (from your home salad bar) Vegetable Stir-Fry Perfect Quinoa (1/2 cup only) with extra olive oil 1 tablespoon Olive Tapenade
Day 4:	Rich Avocado Soup Steamed Broccoli 1 tablespoon Walnut Tapenade 4 celery stalks for dipping the tapenade
Day 5:	Roasted Butternut Squash Soup Brussels Sprout Stir-Fry 1 tablespoon Walnut Tapenade
Day 6:	Los Lobos Vegetable Soup Vegetable Stir-Fry Grilled Asparagus 2 tablespoons Hummus 4 celery stalks for dipping the tapenade or hummus
Day 7:	Roasted Butternut Squash Soup Steamed Broccoli 1 tablespoon Olive Tapenade 1 tablespoon Walnut Tapenade 4 celery stalks for dipping the tapenade

After Your Grow a New Body Program

During the seven-day Grow a New Body program, you will have been eating a reduced calorie and reduced protein diet. As a result, your mTOR signaling will have gone down dramatically, and your body will have entered into repair and regeneration mode.

Now you can introduce a nice serving of protein, such as the fish dish below or poached eggs, to upregulate mTOR and begin building muscle.

Grilled Halibut in Avocado Sauce

2 Servings

This is one of my favorite fish dishes. Try it the day after you finish your program, to up your protein intake. Halibut is a delicate fish that grills very well. You can also prepare this dish in the oven.

For the halibut:

Two 8-ounce halibut steaks

½ teaspoon Himalayan salt

½ teaspoon ground black pepper

1 tablespoon coconut oil

1 lemon cut in half, for garnish

Cilantro, for garnish

For the avocado sauce:

1 ripe avocado, peeled and pitted

¼ cup water or almond milk

¼ cup lemon juice

1 tablespoon chopped green onions

¼ teaspoon smoked paprika, plus a dash for garnish

¼ teaspoon Himalayan salt

¼ teaspoon freshly ground black pepper

Preheat the grill to medium-high heat, around 330°F. Season the fish with a generous amount of salt and pepper, as well as lightly coating the steaks in coconut oil. Grill 4 to 5 minutes per side, until the fish starts to flake.

While the fish is cooking, you can prepare the avocado sauce.

Place the avocado, water (or almond milk), lemon juice, green onions, paprika, salt, and pepper in a blender and puree until smooth. Add more water or almond milk if the puree is too thick.

Make a bed of the avocado sauce, and place the grilled halibut on top. Garnish with fresh cilantro and lemon slices, and sprinkle a dash of paprika over the fish.

Serve with grilled asparagus, steamed broccoli, or Brussels sprouts on the side.

Poached Eggs with Avocado and Chard

2 Servings

Poaching eggs in water is a fabulous way to cook them without exposing the eggs to high heat that can readily destroy many nutrients.

2 tablespoons apple cider vinegar

¼ teaspoon sea salt

2 organic, free-range eggs

1 tablespoon coconut oil

2 leaves chard, chopped

2 cloves garlic, sliced thinly

2 leaves kale, chopped

¼ teaspoon black pepper

1 avocado, sliced, for garnish

1 tablespoon chopped parsley leaves, for garnish

1 tablespoon MCT oil

Pour the vinegar into a saucepan with at least two inches of boiling water. Add a pinch of salt, and then lower the heat to simmer. Stir the simmering water with a spoon to create a small whirlpool. Crack the egg into a cup, and add the egg to the middle of the swirling water. Repeat for the second egg.

Place the coconut oil, chard, garlic, and kale in a frying pan and cook on medium heat for 3 minutes. You can add a few drops of water and cover to steam the greens.

Serve with avocado slices, black pepper, and chopped parsley. Drizzle with MCT oil.

Chapter 18

YOUR LONGEVITY PLAN: PRACTICING PREVENTION

The most important intervention for making sure that your health span equals your life span is nutritional and spiritual. The food you eat and the supplements you take to switch on the longevity genes and upgrade repair systems are by far the most significant. Second are the spiritual practices. The immediate benefit of these is that they heal your emotions, and the unbridled emotions of the limbic brain are the root cause of many diseases.

Until recently humans lived short and brutish lives. The average life span of a man born in London in the 18th century was 34 years of age. So the strongest and the fittest, but fast-aging individuals, got to live to what was then considered a ripe old age, while those genetically predisposed to age slowly did not survive the epidemics, viral infections, malnutrition, and lack of hygiene of the era.

Today with the advances in public health and in medicine, humans are enjoying much longer life spans, and the slow-agers among us are tomorrow's centenarians. But there is a catch to this seemingly great news. While our life span is increasing, our health span remains largely unchanged. Modern medicine has extended the life of convalescence in old age but has done nothing to extend the years where we enjoy good health. So while osteoporosis and a broken hip bone resulted in a more or less rapid decline and death 50 years ago, today with modern medical care we can replace a hip and draw out the period of convalescence for decades.

We do not want to spend an extra 20 or 30 years of life bed-ridden.

Cancer researcher Mikhail V. Blagosklonny observes that "traditional medicine increases number of old people in bad health. However, extension of life span by lengthening only the morbidity phase will make the cost of medical care unsustainable for society. Anti-aging medicine can solve this crisis by delaying the morbidity (deterioration) phase." He proposes that mTOR is the accelerator, that a hyper-accelerated mTOR may increase the chances for survival early in life and successful reproduction, at the expense of accelerated aging.[1]

Blagosklonny explains that animals in the wild do not live very long lives and therefore do not experience aging. An older wildebeest in the African plain quickly becomes food for a young hyena. Therefore, living beings need to grow as fast as possible so that they can produce young, before their eggs and sperm perish from other causes, including predators and malnutrition.

In the young, mTOR is the *growth engine enzyme*. It ensures the survival of the fastest and fittest, and it does so by speeding up the activity of building muscle and bone. The weak and infirm children—those with less active mTOR—frequently died during birth or shortly thereafter from malnutrition. Biologists call this natural selection, where Mother Nature selects only the fittest to survive and pass on their genes to the future. And these survivors had their mTOR engines revved up and red-lining.

Since mTOR is the accelerator of growth during our youth, it is the accelerator of aging. Riding on the horse of mTOR is the metaphorical Angel of Death. This is why it has been called the *aging engine enzyme*. So if we can slow down the activity level of mTOR, we can take nature's foot off of the accelerator of aging and experience a longer health span. We can delay the morbidity phase of life—those terrible last few months or years of our life. And if we are lucky, perhaps we can die from old age, perhaps even in our sleep, the way our ancestors often did.

Today we know how to slow down the mTOR engine.

The only tested strategy that results in increased longevity and health span is caloric restriction (CR), the reduction of caloric intake without malnutrition. For a long time scientists believed that it was the reduction in calories that made a difference, and this meant the reduction of dietary sugars and carbs.

Recent research suggests that CR works because of a reduction of essential amino acids, the components of proteins. It turns out that protein restriction is at the root of the longevity and health benefits of CR!

The presence of certain amino acids, particularly leucine, activates mTOR, which as we mentioned earlier, works at supersonic speeds. Leucine is perhaps the most potent inducer of muscle growth. And we find the highest concentrations of leucine in dairy, meats, and eggs.

It's as if Mother Nature waited for our ancestors to be lucky in their hunt and return home with game to switch on mTOR and put the body into accelerated muscle growth mode, and into reproduction. I had a professor when I was studying anthropology who would say that the myth of the "great white hunter" was a lie, that it was very difficult to hunt game, and that we were not hunters and gatherers but scavengers and gatherers. He would grin and tell the story of a group of Paleolithic guys coming across fresh roadkill by the trailside, shooing away the vultures, and bringing the kill back home and telling their wives, "Look what I caught for you, honey, can we have sex now?"

It was during these times of abundant meat that the young thrived, that mothers had enough iron to endure the feeding of a growing embryo and the blood lost during childbirth. All great for the species to guarantee its long life. But not great for individual longevity.

It turns out that reducing your protein intake can extend longevity, improve metabolic fitness, and increase stress resistance.[2] It's not the carbs, after all! This will be great news for the vegetarians and vegans, who have heard for decades that you cannot get adequate protein from plant sources. Not true.

Turns out that the key to slow aging and postponing of the decrepitude associated with old age is reducing the intake of meats, dairy, and eggs rich in leucine. And you can only lower your levels of leucine by reducing your intake of animal proteins. You would have to consume almost 10 pounds of white cabbage or 100 apples to have the same amount of leucine in a 3 oz steak. In addition, it turns out that plant-derived polyphenols and flavonoids are natural inhibitors of mTOR and help resolve diabetes and obesity.[3]

Perhaps the most potent stimulator of mTOR are dairy products. Think of it, mother's milk is the preferred diet of the newborn infant during the first months of life when babies grow at an extraordinary rate, a growth rate maintained by the activation of mTOR. Milk proteins are beginning-of-life proteins and really not meant for consumption after the first two years of life. And dairy products pack a double whammy, in that they activate mTOR through high leucine concentrations, but they also stimulate the IGF-1 signaling pathway that shuts down cellular detoxification! And while a human mother's milk contains about 1 gram of protein per milliliter, cow milk contains nearly 3.4 grams per milliliter! Cows of course grow much more rapidly (and start walking sooner) than human babies, so they need the additional protein. Humans do not.

Okinawans are one of the healthiest people and among those who live the longest on the planet, living in what are now popularly called *blue zones*, and their diet is only 10 percent protein, most of it coming from plant sources. They eat the equivalent of one egg and one piece of fish per month. Their longevity is surpassed only by the lacto-ovo vegetarian Adventists in Loma Linda, California, who live on average seven years longer than their California neighbors.

What You Can Do to Protect Your Health

Remove your amalgams. If you have mercury fillings in your mouth, take them out. These fillings leach mercury into your systems, and mercury is a neurotoxin. Be sure that you go to a biological dentist, and that this is not the first time he or she is trying to do this procedure. Amalgam removal must be done with great care, using aspirators and rubber dams. The day you are set to remove your amalgams, drink an eight-ounce glass of water with chlorella powder dissolved in it, to bind any mercury that leaks into your stomach. Take a bottle of water with lots of chlorella in it and rinse your mouth with your water whenever your dentist tells you to rinse. And after leaving the office, drink another eight-ounce glass of chlorella water. The European Parliament has banned the use of mercury fillings in Europe after 2023.

Consider heavy metal chelation. We were never exposed to heavy metals until very recently. All the mercury we encountered was bound into rocks and not free in the atmosphere (in the form of methylmercury) from burning coal for fuel or in large ocean fish like tuna. Aluminum use is widespread, from aluminum foil to the coffee pods for use in espresso machines to deodorant. Lead exposure comes from lead plumbing (do you remember living in a house with lead pipes?). Arsenic is found in pesticides and in all rice, even the organic brands, because rice is grown in flooded fields, and arsenic binds to the young rice shoots. I like the Andy Cutler protocol that you can do at home. It is safe and proven. The Europeans (the Germans in particular) are far ahead of their American counterparts in heavy metal chelation. If you do IV chelation, be sure you work with a knowledgeable physician. I work with Petra Kscheschinski, a mitochondrial medicine practitioner near Freiburg, Germany.

Prevent Cancer

One of every two men and one of three women will develop a serious cancer at some point in their lives. This is not the benign skin cancers we are all susceptible to, these are serious cancers requiring cut, burn, or kill treatment. While cancer is almost unheard of among hunter-gatherers, or in societies that have not adopted the Western diet and lifestyle, it is rampant in the developed world. All of us have a relative who is struggling with a cancer or died from it.

But there are ways that we can lower our risk for developing cancer, and strategies we can employ to help ourselves to heal if we have been diagnosed. Here they are:

Enhance your body's ability to burn fat. A ketogenic diet and/or fasting is a key strategy for preventing cancer. Remember that cancer cells have reverted back to a more primitive state and are unable to burn fats efficiently. They can only thrive when in the presence of abundant carbohydrates (sugars). Drs. Rainer J. Klement and Ulrike Kämmerer at the Department of Radiation Oncology, University Hospital of Würzburg, in Germany, have found that by "systematically reducing the amount of dietary carbohydrates (CHOs) one could suppress, or at least delay, the emergence of cancer, and that proliferation of already existing tumor cells could be slowed down."

How elegant. You cut off the tumor cells' energy supply, and they begin to die. The authors state that "contrary to normal cells, most malignant cells depend on steady glucose availability in the blood for their energy and biomass generating demands and are not able to metabolize significant amounts of fatty acids or ketone bodies due to mitochondrial dysfunction."[4]

If you have been diagnosed with cancer, or if there is a high incidence of cancer in your family, it is essential that you sign on to a ketogenic diet and the intermittent fasting described in this book.

The next key strategy to prevent cancer is to **detoxify your body and brain.** Begin by getting a whole-house water filter that eliminates chlorine and fluoride. You get more than three times more toxins from the water you shower and bathe with than from the water you drink.

In Russia scientists are finding that some cancer tumors are loaded with heavy metals, and that perhaps this is the body's attempt at eliminating these. Be sure that you have removed the mercury from your mouth (the "silver" fillings) and that you do a heavy metal "push test" where you take an oral chelator to determine your body's load of mercury, lead, arsenic, and others.

Above all, remember that prevention is the key.

Prevent Heart Disease

A heart attack occurs when blood flow to a region of your heart is blocked, usually by a clot formed in a ruptured blood vessel. Every year one million Americans suffer heart attacks, and more people die from heart attacks than from any other kind of disease. Yet cardiologists believe that 90 percent of heart attacks can be prevented through diet and lifestyle changes.[5]

The key is to avoid trans fats, which are often hiding under the label of hydrogenated oils. Trans fats increase the small LDL cholesterol that builds up plaque in your arteries. Sugars, carbs, and processed foods increase the levels of small LDL cholesterol particles.

Saturated fats, once thought to be evil, actually increase the large, harmless LDL cholesterol. So you want to eat a lot of fresh vegetables, not overcooked. Organic, grass-fed butter and meats. Pastured eggs. Raw nuts and seeds. Coconut oil. Olive oil. Nut butters.

Berries are at the top of my list. The more colors the better. Researchers at Harvard found that persons who eat a significant amount of fruit daily lower their risk for heart disease by nearly 30 percent.[6] But be careful with the very sweet fruits, and remember that eating a watermelon is like eating a popsicle, as it is full of sugar with no fiber.

Prevent Alzheimer's and Dementia

Today there are nearly 50 million people with dementia, a condition that was largely unheard of a century ago. There is nothing as frightening as the thought of losing one's mind, or not remembering the names of your loved ones.

In some circles Alzheimer's is being called type 3 diabetes because of its connection to high blood sugar and a sugar-rich diet. And today we know that the foods that increase inflammation, including processed grains and refined carbs, are a risk factor for developing Alzheimer's. The statistics for this disease are terrifying. They show that if you live to be 85 years old, you will have a 50 percent risk of having diagnosable Alzheimer's.

Today you can count on living to 100 years old, barring unforeseen accidents. So how do we skew the odds in our favor? How do we prevent the dementias?

The food you eat is not only the cause, but also the cure. I have been speaking about it throughout the book. Avoid the sugars, restrict the carbs, limit the protein intake to primarily plant-based protein sources, and eat healthy fats. Here is what else you can do.

Take vitamin D3. Researchers followed 50 patients at risk of Parkinson's disease (PD) for nearly 30 years and found that the risk for PD among those patients that had the highest levels of vitamin D3 were nearly 75 percent lower than for patients lacking this essential vitamin.[7] They concluded that vitamin D3 appears to be neuroprotective and can prevent the onset of PD.

The reason you have not heard of this study published in the *Archives of Neurology* is that you cannot patent vitamin D3. No pharmaceutical company is going to invest in long-term clinical trials on a vitamin you can buy over the counter for 20 cents, but that reduces your risk for PD by 75 percent!

Take DHA. Another study published in the *Archives of Neurology* showed that persons who have the highest level of plasma DHA, our favorite omega-3 fatty acid, had an 85 percent reduced risk of developing Alzheimer's.[8] Again, no drug company worth their salt is going to sponsor a long-term study costing millions of dollars to test if a fish-oil tablet that costs 50 cents can help prevent this devastating condition.

Exercise regularly and engage in physical activity. A study by Dr. Kirk Eriksen at UCLA and his colleagues at the University of Pittsburgh School of Medicine showed that regular aerobic exercise, regardless of the person's age, reduced the risk for Alzheimer's by 50 percent.[9]

The 5 Most Important Blood Tests You Can Get

Extraordinarily sensitive blood tests today allow you to detect changes in your body and correct imbalances that can lead to disease. I get these tests on a yearly basis and review them with my doctor.

1. CBC (complete blood count): A low-cost blood panel that offers you an eagle's vision of your health and can indicate the presence of infection, anemia, cholesterol, blood glucose, and critical minerals. It will take a little time to become familiar with the results. Note that the optimal ranges are different from the laboratory reference ranges.

Optimal ranges[10]:

Glucose	70–85 mg/dl
Cholesterol	180–200 mg/dl
LDL	Under 100 mg/dl
HDL	Over 55 mg/dl
Triglycerides	Under 100 mg/dl

2. C-Reactive Protein: Inflammation is the cause of and is associated with every major medical condition. C-reactive protein is a sensitive marker of inflammation, and one that responds fairly rapidly (in a matter of days) to lifestyle and dietary interventions. It is a reliable predictor of coronary heart disease.

Optimal ranges:

Men	<0.55 mg/L
Women	<1.5 mg/L

3. Hemoglobin A1C: This test measures your glucose levels over the last two to three months, and it is a reliable predictor of heart disease in persons with or without diabetes. High blood sugar and inflammation is the perfect cancer environment. This test will show you how fertile your inner environment is for cancer and other pathology.

Optimal ranges: <4.5%

4. Homocysteine: This is an amino acid that is formed as the body metabolizes sulfur-containing methionine. High levels of homocysteine are associated with an increased risk of heart attacks and bone fractures, including hip fractures, as well as reduced cognitive performance.

Optimal ranges: <7.2 µmol/L

5. IGF-1: This hormone, along with growth hormone, helps to regulate the growth of bone and other tissues during our youth. Later in life we want to be sure to have a low level of IGF-1, given that we do not need any additional arms or fingers. We have explained how IGF-1 is a signaling molecule that switches on and off the cellular repair and recycling programs. IGF-1 is primarily a protein nutrient sensor (amino acids); and red meat, fish, and seafood will increase our levels of IGF-1, which are associated with an increased level of heart disease and cancer.

IGF-1 is also a cancer tumor marker. There are no absolute reference ranges for IGF-1, so it's best used to gauge how well you are responding to the Grow a New Body program. I find that levels of this tumor marker will drop between 30 and 50 percent within a week of starting the program. This is an inexpensive test, and gives you measurable feedback as to how well your body is eliminating cellular waste and switching on the longevity genes.

I tell my students that prevention is like changing the oil in your car, while treatment is like changing the engine. Our health-care systems do not invest in prevention. Coronary artery bypass graft, known among surgeons as "cabbage," is a $50,000 procedure—and the most frequently performed surgery in the United States. When an artery gets clogged, heart surgeons cut out a piece of the artery and replace it with new pipes, much like a city does with aging water mains. It has a terrible success rate, as vascular disease is a systemic condition and not limited to a few inches of artery. Furthermore, this is a condition that is readily prevented through diet or that can be treated cheaply and effectively with chelating agents.

I invite you to take charge of the experiment in longevity and health that we are all taking part in. We can make the wise choices that will lead to long health and vibrant lives by practicing prevention and having the experience of Oneness!

CONCLUSION

ONE SPIRIT MEDICINE AND BEYOND

We shall not cease from exploration
And the end of all our exploring
Will be to arrive where we started
And know the place for the first time.

— FROM "LITTLE GIDDING," BY T. S. ELIOT

The future Buddha had to face many tests. As soon as he sat under the Bodhi Tree, he was approached by the demon-god Mara, the lord of death, with weapons in hand, surrounded by his army. Legend has it that all the protecting deities of the universe fled, terrified, yet Siddhartha remained unmoved. Even though the demon hurled thunderbolts and flaming arrows at him, they were transformed into flowers that landed at Siddhartha's feet. Finally, the future Buddha reached down with his right hand to touch the ground, and the earth goddess herself appeared to bear witness to his illumination. With a mighty roar, she drove away the demon-god.

The lore says that in the long night leading to his enlightenment, the Buddha acquired three gifts: the divine eye of omniscient vision and knowledge of all his previous existences; the understanding of karma and the chain of causality and release, or liberation; and the Four Noble Truths, the fundamental laws of existence. It is said that the Buddha considered keeping this wisdom to himself, doubting that humans were ready for such a teaching, but Brahma intervened, persuading him to share with men and gods the profound truths that he had discovered.

What do we do after receiving One Spirit Medicine? Do we, like the Buddha, go into the world and teach what we've learned? Do we long to escape the battlefield altogether, like Arjuna, distraught that we can't prevent the suffering of life, and retreat from problems we see? Or, "like most of the rest of us," as Joseph Campbell puts it, do we "invent a false, finally unjustified, image of oneself as an exceptional phenomenon in the world, not guilty as others are, but justified in one's inevitable sinning because one represents the good. Such self-righteousness leads to a misunderstanding, not only of oneself but of the nature of both man and the cosmos."[1]

The heroes and heroines—both mythic and real—whose journeys we have explored throughout these pages remind us that our goal is to establish a relationship with the universal guiding principle we call One Spirit. And then we can set about repairing the torn fabric of our own lives, our health, and our humanity, which is sorely in need of any wisdom we can share.

Healing the World

So how, then, do we bring our gifts to the world? The global situation is increasingly disquieting on every level—political, economic, social, and environmental. The first decade of the 21st century was the hottest in recorded history. In 2007, climate experts told us that to avoid irreversible consequences, we would have to make sure the level of carbon dioxide in the atmosphere did not exceed 350 parts per million (ppm). But by 2014, we had already passed 400 ppm with no sign of slowing down. Biologists, directly linking the rate of animal and plant species extinction to greenhouse gas emissions, warn that we're on the brink of mass extinction. Mass extinctions have occurred only five times since life emerged on Earth some 3.5 billion years ago. Now we're facing the sixth such catastrophic event.

When we're stuck in our old paradigms and beliefs, we assume that as individuals we're helpless to save the whales or the planet or humanity. It's true: none of us alone can halt terrorism, wipe out environmental toxins, stop the melting of the polar ice caps, or avert economic crisis. What we can do, however, is heal from the sicknesses that threaten our survival. We can heal our inner masculine, giving up violence as a way to resolve conflict. We can heal our inner feminine, becoming stewards of the earth. And we've learned that with Spirit and one another, we are continually co-creating the world. We can always do a better job.

The Grow a New Body program enhances the body's ability to eliminate toxins we're exposed to, whether they're pollutants in the air or water or our food or the mental poisons of unhealthy thinking and belief systems. It also allows us to upgrade the brain so that it supports the consciousness that creates health. And the bonus is that in helping ourselves, we also help the earth. As we discard toxic and predatory beliefs and behaviors, we can participate in co-creating a sustainable way for everyone to live together on the planet.

As the Lakota Sioux phrase *Mitakuye Oyasin*—"All my relations"—implies, we're all connected, we're all in this together. Recovery is reciprocal: heal yourself, heal the world; heal the world, heal yourself. Once you're dedicated to improving your own health and the health of the earth and all her creatures, the Spirit world will rally behind you to support your commitment.

Inner Harmony

Peace and harmony in the world begin with your inner world. Your gut is a world unto itself—an immensely complex ecosystem. And learning to live harmoniously with the microbes inside you is clearly crucial to your survival. Sustainable health depends on learning to not just survive but to thrive, in collaboration with all the bacteria, viruses, and other cells in your body.

Your body is your earth, the ground that your life rests on. Dumping noxious pharmaceuticals into it is shortsighted. We're now facing deadly bacterial outbreaks because of our overuse of antibiotics and antimicrobial cleansers, which has allowed ever-resourceful microbes to mutate into drug-resistant strains. Your health and the health of the planet rest on forging a new relationship with all creatures, including the microbes in your body and the mitochondria in your cells.

From Stewards to Dreamers

Historically, the Abrahamic religions—Christianity, Judaism, and Islam—have privileged man over nature. To this way of thinking, our earthly home is merely a way station we stop at on our way to the bliss of eternal life. Taking care of the planet and all its creatures has been largely left to chance—not humanity's responsibility, at any rate. To scientists, however, the need to assume care of the earth is more pressing. Most agree that we're overtaxing the planet and that it's up to us to make the tough political and economic choices we've been deferring to future generations.

After years of doing research in aboriginal cultures, I'm very aware of how much the indigenous worldview differs from the scientific paradigm of the West. To the indigenous, the welfare of the planet comes first. That includes the well-being of all the earth's inhabitants equally, nonhuman and human alike. Indigenous people believe we must take care of the planet not because it is a temporary home granted to us by a distant God but because it's Mother Earth herself—our permanent home, into which we are reborn lifetime after lifetime.

As Krishna tells Arjuna:

> *Even as a person casts off worn-out clothes and puts on others that are new, so the embodied Self casts off worn-out bodies and enters into others that are new. . . . Weapons cut It not; fire burns It not; water wets It not; the wind does not wither It. . . . This Self cannot be cut nor burnt nor wetted nor withered. . . . Eternal, all-pervading, unchanging, immovable, the Self is the same forever.*[2]

Earth is the heaven we earn after a long journey through the Spirit realms, and we must tend it as our Eden. Otherwise, the planet may decide it is unsustainable to continue supporting the greediest of her children. And because we the greediest have commandeered most of the resources for our own use, we've put the rest of nature—the innocent—in jeopardy.

For the healing and survival of Earth, we need a new dream now.

Choosing Evolution

Despite all the devastation we've wrought to the earth, however, there are hopeful signs. All around the globe, people are creating new forms to replace the old ones that have crumbled beyond repair, whether in infrastructure, government, the economy, health care, or social welfare. Institutions are adapting in response to current needs, and so are our bodies and our brains.

Adaptation refers to short-term changes in individuals or groups to make them better suited to their environment. In times of stress and global crisis like the present, we may become ill—or we may become extraordinarily healthy, if we learn to adapt and thrive in rapidly changing conditions. Compared to adaptation, evolution—long-term genetic change to ensure survival of the species—moves at a glacial pace. But there's evidence now that our physiology is about to make an evolutionary leap. Over the past couple of centuries, the human brain has been steadily shrinking in size, losing some 10 percent of its volume,[3] a cluster of neurons about the size of a tennis ball. In evolutionary terms, this is a dramatic change, and a prelude to what's known as quantum speciation, the leap that can occur when a species is threatened with extinction.

We're at an evolutionary threshold. In the past, we ensured our survival by killing off competing species—or in the case of the Neanderthals, our distant relatives. And we've decimated or obliterated more than a few furry, finned, or feathered species. A new evolutionary leap might allow our species to survive, but we can't make the leap using the archaic methods of the tyrant-king brain. We can only make it with the creative resources available to us from the higher brain.

A Different Brain

The jungle is a noisy place, and so is the virtual world of the Internet and social media. Undoubtedly the future belongs to those who are adapted to the virtual world—who are at home in the virtual jungle and aware of which snapping twigs to listen to and which to ignore.

The generation coming of age now was raised in a totally wired world. They've used technology to communicate since they were old enough to tap out a message on a digital screen. Today, e-mail, cell phones, online forums, and social media are the dominant ways we engage with one another on everything that matters in our lives, from supporting efforts to reduce the causes of global poverty to making plans with our friends for Saturday night. Now, every generation needs to be able to move between the virtual world and the world of the senses as easily as the jaguar moves between the visible and invisible realms.

Mother Earth is humanity's home, and we are charged with being her stewards.

Out of Chaos Comes Creation

The shamans believe that long ago, in the invisible world, the blueprint of creation was drawn. Chaos was turned into order, into the cosmos, through the actions of courageous beings who were able to dream new worlds into being, in much the same way gamers are creating virtual worlds today. Our Earth was dreamed into being with the perfect conditions to sustain life, with steady temperatures in the narrow band between the freezing and boiling points of water.

Just as life on Earth began in a primordial soup, today we again find ourselves in a primordial soup of creative potential. From that perspective we can turn chaos into order and beauty. Healing is one form of order. When we bring greater order and harmony to the body, illness disappears, and we recover. We create the conditions for health, and disease goes away.

The biggest breakthroughs in brain science today are neuroplasticity—the brain's ability to change and adapt, forming new neural connections in response to our experiences and environmental demands—and epigenetics, changes in the way genes are expressed. From Chapter 3, Dethroning the Tyrant King, you now know that you can rewire your brain for cooperation and joy instead of competition and fear. And from Chapter 6, Superfoods and Super Supplements, you know that you can use a phytonutrient-rich diet to rebalance the microorganisms in your gut, creating health and mental clarity, and affecting your gene expression. Within this lifetime, you can actually experience a new body—the "new suit of clothes" that the Bhagavad Gita speaks about. Neuroplasticity and epigenetics tell us we don't have to suffer the illnesses of our ancestors or perpetuate their beliefs. We can experience states of physical well-being and mental acuity that we never thought possible, and wisdom we never imagined. And we can find peace.

The quest for inner peace may be one of the most fundamental human longings. There's a famous story about a seeker who comes to the Ch'an Buddhist master Bodhidharma and begs the great teacher to pacify his soul. "Bring me your soul, and I will pacify it," Bodhidharma tells him. "That's the problem," the speaker says. "I have looked for years, but I cannot find it." With that, Bodhidharma declares, "Your wish is granted." The seeker understands and leaves in peace.

What the seeker realizes is that the soul, the fundamental truth of who we are, isn't something separate from the body. It isn't something "out there" that can be found. As Joseph Campbell explains it, "Those who know not only that the Everlasting lives in them but that what they, and all things really are, *is* the Everlasting, dwell in the groves of the wish-fulfilling trees, drink the brew of immortality, and listen everywhere to the unheard music of eternal concord."[4]

Reach out and take the fruit of the tree of life that is within your grasp!

APPENDIX

Creating Your Longevity Spa

At Los Lobos Spa in Chile, we have state-of-the-art technology for supporting the process of growing a new body. I am going to share with you a few devices that you may want to invest in that will make a huge difference in your health.

Not everyone can afford the expense of equipping a home spa with devices that will help you protect your health and support longevity. If you are a health practitioner (or a health fanatic like me), you may want to consider outfitting your home spa or professional office with the following equipment.

Far-infrared (FIR) sauna: This is a must. A FIR sauna helps lower inflammation, burn body fat, boost metabolism, and improves mitochondrial function. I have a FIR sauna in my office and one at home. Whereas a conventional sauna heats up the surface of your skin, a FIR sauna's rays will penetrate up to three centimeters into the skin to help you detoxify from endogenous and environmental pollutants. This is one of the best investments you can make in your health.

Interval hypoxia-hyperoxia training (IHHT): This device, manufactured by Cell Gym in Germany, regulates the concentration of oxygen you receive via a face mask. In effect, the instrument takes you from the beach (high oxygen concentration) to the top of Mount Everest (low oxygen, hypoxia) every six minutes. As a result, the weak mitochondria in your body are oxygen starved and begin to die off. Intermittent hypoxia stimulates the Nrf2 pathway and switches on the longevity genes, as well as the natural antioxidant production inside every cell. This is one of the best investments I have ever made, as it triggers the production of new, healthy mitochondria. Website is https://cellgym.de.

Ozone therapy: Physicians in Europe have been employing ozone therapy for over 50 years. Ozone works by switching on the Nrf2 detox pathway and activating antioxidant enzymes and free-radical scavengers. We administer ozone treatments rectally using a small catheter. A 100 ml syringe is loaded with ozone gas and infused into the body over a three-minute period, and the procedure is repeated with another 100 ml. I use equipment by Humares in Germany, who have been manufacturing medical-grade devices for decades. If you are going to get a device for your personal use, be sure to get a quality product that delivers clean, precise doses. This is one of the most important prevention and longevity instruments. Website is http://humares.de.

ENDNOTES

Introduction

1. Roman Thaler et al., "Anabolic and Antiresorptive Modulation of Bone Homeostasis by the Epigenetic Modulator Sulforaphane, a Naturally Occurring Isothiocyanate," *Journal of Biological Chemistry* 291 (March 2016): 6754–6771. DOI: 10.1074/jbc.M115.678235.

2. "Risk Factors," Alzheimer's Association, http://www.alz.org/alzheimers_disease_causes_risk_factors.asp.

3. "FastStats: Obesity and Overweight," Centers for Disease Control and Prevention, updated May 14, 2014, http://www.cdc.gov/nchs/fastats/obesity-overweight.htm.

4. M. Kivipelto et al., "The Finnish Geriatric Intervention Study to Prevent Cognitive Impairment and Disability (FINGER): Study Design and Progress," *Alzheimer's & Dementia* 9, no. 6 (November 2013): 657–65. DOI: 10.1016/j.jalz.2012.09.012.

Chapter 1

1. Raj Chetty et al., "The Association Between Income and Life Expectancy in the United States, 2001–2014," *Journal of the American Medical Association* 315, no. 16 (April 26, 2016): 1750–1766. DOI: 10.1001/jama.2016.4226.

Chapter 3

1. Wei-Yi Ong et al., "Protective Effects of Ginseng on Neurological Disorders," *Frontiers in Aging Neuroscience* 7, no. 129 (July 2015). DOI: 10.3389/fnagi.2015.00129.

2. Jared Diamond, "The Worst Mistake in the History of the Human Race (from the May 1987 issue)," *Discover Magazine*, May 1, 1999, http://discovermagazine.com/1987/may/02-the-worst-mistake-in-the-history-of-the-human-race.

3. Vincent J. Felitti et al., "Relationship of Childhood Abuse and Household Dysfunction to Many of the Leading Causes in Death in Adults: The Adverse Childhood Experiences (ACE) Study," *American Journal of Preventive Medicine* 14, no. 4 (May 1998): 245–258.

4. Bogdan Draganski et al., "Temporal and Spatial Dynamics of Brain Structure Changes during Extensive Learning," *Journal of Neuroscience* 26, no. 23 (June 7, 2006): 6314–6317.

Chapter 4

1. "The Medicare Prescription Drug Benefit Fact Sheet," Kaiser Family Foundation, September 19, 2014, http://www.kaiseredu.org/Issue-Modules/Prescription-Drug-Costs/Background-Brief.aspx.

2. Kathrin Endt et al., "The Microbiota Mediates Pathogen Clearance from the Gut Lumen after Non-Typhoidal *Salmonella* Diarrhea," *PLOS Pathogens* 6, no. 9 (September 9, 2010), https://doi.org/10.1371/journal.ppat.1001097.

3. United States Department of Agriculture, "Profiling Food Consumption in America," chap. 2 in *Agriculture Fact Book, 2001–2002* (Washington, DC: U.S. Government Printing Office, 2003), 20.

4. Owen Dyer, "Is Alzheimer's Really Just Type III Diabetes?," *National Review of Medicine* 2, no. 21 (December 15, 2005), http://www.nationalreviewofmedicine.com/issue/2005/12_15/2_advances_medicine01_21.html.

5. Magalie Lenoir et al., "Intense Sweetness Surpasses Cocaine Reward," *PLoS One* 2, no. 8 (2007): e698. DOI: 10.1371/journal.pone.0000698.

6. Kokab Namkin, Mahmood Zardast, and Fatemeh Basirinejad, "*Saccharomyces boulardii* in *Helicobacter pylori* Eradication in Children: A Randomized Trial from Iran," *Iranian Journal of Pediatrics* 26, no. 1 (February 2016): e3768. DOI: 10.5812/ijp.3768.

7. C. Costalos et al., "Enteral Feeding of Premature Infants with *Saccharomyces boulardii*," *Early Human Development* 74, no. 2 (November 2003): 89–96. PMID: 14580749.

8. Lund University, "Estrogen in Birth Control Pills Has a Negative Impact on Fish," ScienceDaily, March 4, 2016, www.sciencedaily.com/releases/2016/03/160304092230.htm.

9. Chia-Yu Chang, Der-Shin Ke, and Jen-Yin Chen, "Essential Fatty Acids and Human Brain," *Acta Neurologica Taiwanica* 18, no. 4 (December 2009): 231–241. PMID: 20329590.

10. Vazquez et al., "Intragastric and Intraperitoneal Administration of Cry1Ac Protoxin from *Bacillus thuringiensis* Induces Systemic and Mucosal Antibody Responses in Mice," *Life Sciences* 64, no. 21 (1999): 1897–1912.

11. A. Aris and S. Leblanc, "Maternal and Fetal Exposure to Pesticides Associated to Genetically Modified Foods in Eastern Townships of Quebec, Canada," *Reproductive Toxicology* 31, no. 4 (May 2011): 528–33. DOI: 10.1016/j.reprotox.2011.02.004.

12. A. Fasano, "Zonulin and Its Regulation of Intestinal Barrier Function: The Biological Door to Inflammation, Autoimmunity, and Cancer," *Physiological Reviews* 91, no. 1 (Jan 2011): 151–75. DOI: 10.1152/physrev.00003.2008.

13. Henry C. Lin, "Small Intestinal Bacterial Overgrowth: A Framework for Understanding Irritable Bowel Syndrome," *Journal of the American Medical Association* 292, no. 7 (August 18, 2004): 852–858.

14. Els van Nood et al., "Duodenal Infusion of Donor Feces for Recurrent *Clostridium difficile*," *New England Journal of Medicine* 368, no. 5 (January 31, 2013): 407–415.

Chapter 5

1. Ioannis Delimaris, "Adverse Effects Associated with Protein Intake above the Recommended Dietary Allowance for Adults," *ISRN Nutrition* 2013, (June 2013), Article ID 126929. DOI: 10.5402/2013/126929.

2. M N Corradetti and K-L Guan, "Upstream of the Mammalian Target of Rapamycin: Do All Roads Pass Through mTOR?" *Oncogene* 25 (16 October 2006): 6347–6360. DOI: 10.1038/sj.onc.1209885.

3. Luigi Fontana et al., "Long-Term Effects of Calorie or Protein Restriction on Serum IGF-1 and IGFBP-3 Concentration in Humans," *Aging Cell* 7, no. 5 (October 2008): 681–687. DOI: 10.1111/j.1474-9726.2008.00417.x.

4. Roberto Zoncu, Alejo Efeyan, and David M. Sabatini, "mTOR: From Growth Signal Integration to Cancer, Diabetes and Ageing," *Nature Reviews Molecular Cell Biology* 12, no. 1 (January 2011): 21–35. DOI: 10.1038/nrm3025.

5. Luigi Fontana et al., "Decreased Consumption of Branched Chain Amino Acids Improves Metabolic Health," *Cell Reports* 16, no. 2 (July 12, 2016): 520–530. DOI: 10.1016/j.celrep.2016.05.092.

6. Chia-Wei Cheng et al., "Prolonged Fasting Reduces IGF-1/PKA to Promote Hematopoietic-Stem-Cell-Based Regeneration and Reverse Immunosuppression," *Cell Stem Cell* 13, no. 6 (June 5, 2014): 810–823. https://www.sciencedirect.com/science/article/pii/S1934590914001519.

7. Suzanne Wu, "Fasting Triggers Stem Cell Regeneration of Damaged, Old Immune System," USC News, June 5, 2014, https://news.usc.edu/63669/fasting-triggers-stem-cell-regeneration-of-damaged-old-immune-system/.

8. Marwan A. Maalouf, Jong M. Rho, and Mark P. Mattson, "The Neuroprotective Properties of Calorie Restriction, the Ketogenic Diet, and Ketone Bodies," *Brain Research Reviews* 59, no. 2 (March 2009): 293–315. DOI: 10.1016/j.brainresrev.2008.09.002.

9. Penny Kris-Etherton et al., "AHA Science Advisory: Lyon Diet Heart Study. Benefits of a Mediterranean-Style, National Cholesterol Education Program/American Heart Association Step I Dietary Pattern on Cardiovascular Disease," *Circulation* 103, no. 13 (April 3, 2001): 1823–1825.

Chapter 6

1. Hervé Vaucheret and Yves Chupeau, "Ingested Plant miRNAs Regulate Gene Expression in Animals," *Cell Research* 22, no. 1 (January 2012): 3–5.

2. Jo Robinson, "Breeding the Nutrition Out of Our Food," *New York Times*, May 25, 2013, http://www.nytimes.com/2013/05/26/opinion/sunday/breeding-the-nutrition-out-of-our-food.html?smid=pl-share.

3. Kaitlyn N. Lewis, James Mele, John D. Hayes, and Rochelle Buffenstein, "Nrf2, a Guardian of Healthspan and Gatekeeper of Species Longevity," *Integrative and Comparative Biology* 50, no. 5 (November 2010): 829–843. DOI: 10.1093/icb/icq034.

4. Britta Harbaum et al., "Identification of Flavonoids and Hydroxycinnamic Acids in Pak Choi Varieties (*Brassica campestris* L. ssp. *chinensis* var. *communis*) by HPLC-ESI-MSn and NMR and Their Quantification by HPLC-DAD," *Journal of Agricultural and Food Chemistry* 55, no. 20 (October 3, 2007): 8251–8260.

5. Haitao Luo et al., "Kaempferol Inhibits Angiogenesis and VEGF Expression through Both HIF Dependent and Independent Pathways in Human Ovarian Cancer Cells," *Nutrition and Cancer* 61, no. 4 (2009): 554–563.

6. Morgan E. Levine et al., "Low Protein Intake Is Associated with a Major Reduction in IGF-1, Cancer, and Overall Mortality in the 65 and Younger but Not Older Population," *Cell Metabolism* 19, no. 3 (March 2014): 407–417. DOI: 10.1016/j.cmet.2014.02.006.

7. Thanks to Larry Furtsch of the American Museum of Natural History for this information.

8. Sally Fallon and Mary G. Enig, Ph.D., "Lacto-Fermentation," The Weston A. Price Foundation, January 1, 2000, http://www.westonaprice.org/food-features/lacto-fermentation.

9. Elizabeth P. Ryan et al., "Rice Bran Fermented with *Saccharomyces boulardii* Generates Novel Metabolite Profiles with Bioactivity," *Journal of Agricultural and Food Chemistry* 59, no. 5 (March 9, 2011): 1862–1870. DOI: 10.1021/jf1038103.

10. Martha Clare Morris, Sc.D., et al., "Consumption of Fish and N-3 Fatty Acids and Risk of Incident Alzheimer Disease," *Archives of Neurology* 60, no. 7 (July 2003): 940–946.

11. J. S. Buell, Ph.D., et al., "25-Hydroxyvitamin D, Dementia, and Cerebrovascular Pathology in Elders Receiving Home Services," *Neurology* 74, no. 1 (January 5, 2010): 18–26.

12. Michael F. Holick, M.D., Ph.D., "Vitamin D Deficiency," *New England Journal of Medicine* 357, no. 3 (July 19, 2007): 266–281.

Chapter 7

1. Joyce C. McCann and Bruce N. Ames, "Vitamin K, an Example of Triage Theory: Is Micronutrient Inadequacy Linked to Diseases of Aging?" *The American Journal of Clinical Nutrition* 90, no. 4 (1 October 2009): 889–907. DOI: 10.3945/ajcn.2009.27930.

2. John Neustadt and Steve R. Pieczenik, "Medication-Induced Mitochondrial Damage and Disease," *Molecular Nutrition & Food Research* 52, no. 7 (July 2008): 780.

3. Reiner J. Klement and Ulrike Kämmerer, "Is There a Role for Carbohydrate Restriction in the Treatment and Prevention of Cancer?," *Nutrition & Metabolism* 8, no. 75 (October 2011), http://www.nutritionandmetabolism.com/content/pdf/1743-7075-8-75.pdf.

4. George F. Cahill and Richard L. Veech, "Ketoacids? Good Medicine?," *Transactions of the American Clinical and Climatological Association* 114 (2003): 149–163.

5. W. F. Stewart et al., "Risk of Alzheimer's Disease and Duration of NSAID Use," *Neurology* 48, no. 3 (March 1997): 626–632. PMID: 9065537.

6. H. Chen et al., "Nonsteroidal Anti-inflammatory Drugs and the Risk of Parkinson's Disease," *Annals of Neurology* 58, no. 6 (December 2005): 963–967. DOI: 10.1002/ana.20682.

Chapter 8

1. Jill Bolte Taylor, Ph.D., *My Stroke of Insight: A Brain Scientist's Personal Journey* (New York: Viking Penguin, 2008), 146.

2. Richard Horton, "Offline: What Is Medicine's 5 Sigma?," *Lancet* 385, no. 9976 (April 11, 2015): 1380. DOI: 10.1016/S0140-6736(15)60696-1.

3. Douglas Dean and John Mihalasky, *Executive ESP* (Englewood Cliffs, NJ: Prentice-Hall, 1974).

4. Daniel Kahneman, *Thinking, Fast and Slow* (New York: Farrar, Straus and Giroux, 2011), 11.

5. Peter Gray, Ph.D., "The Decline of Play and Rise in Children's Mental Disorders," *Psychology Today*, January 26, 2010, http://www.psychologytoday.com/blog/freedom-learn/201001/the-decline-play-and-rise-in-childrens-mental-disorders; "Any Mental Illness (AMI) among Adults," National Institute of Mental Health, http://www.nimh.nih.gov/statistics/1ANY-DIS_adult.shtml; "Major Depression among Adults," National Institute of Mental Health, http://www.nimh.nih.gov/health/statistics/prevalence/major-depression-among-adults.shtml; "Any Anxiety Disorder among Adults," National Institute of Mental Health, http://www.nimh.nih.gov/health/statistics/prevalence/any-anxiety-disorder-among-adults.shtml.

6. Jean M. Twenge et al., "Birth Cohort Increases in Psychopathology among Young Americans, 1938–2007: A Cross-Temporal Meta-analysis of the MMPI," *Clinical Psychology Review* 30, no. 2 (March 2010): 152.

7. William J. Broad, "Seeker, Doer, Giver, Ponderer," *New York Times*, July 7, 2014, D1.

Chapter 9

1. Carl Jung, "The Concept of the Collective Unconscious," in *The Portable Jung*, ed. Joseph Campbell (New York: Viking Penguin, 1971), 60.

Chapter 11

1. Rainer J. Klement and Ulrike Kämmerer, "Is There a Role for Carbohydrate Restriction in the Treatment and Prevention of Cancer?," *Nutrition & Metabolism* 8, no. 75 (October 2011), http://www.nutritionandmetabolism.com/content/pdf/1743-7075-8-75.pdf.

Chapter 12

1. Stephen Mitchell, *Bhagavad Gita: A New Translation* (New York: Three Rivers Press, 2000), 95.

2. Mitchell, *Bhadavad Gita*, 21.

3. Mitchell, *Bhadavad Gita*, 88.

Chapter 13

1. Marta Alda et al., "Zen Meditation, Length of Telomeres, and the Role of Experiential Avoidance and Compassion," *Mindfulness* 7, no. 3 (June 2016): 651–659. DOI: 10.1007/s12671-016-0500-5.

2. *The Essential Rumi*, trans. Coleman Barks with John Moyne (San Francisco: HarperSanFrancisco, 1995), 30.

3. "Nagara Sutta: The City," Sutta Nipata 12:65, trans. Thanissaro Bhikkhu (1997), http://www.accesstoinsight.org/tipitaka/sn/sn12/sn12.065.than.html.

4. Chögyam Trungpa, *The Truth of Suffering and the Path of Liberation*, ed. Judith L. Lief (Boston: Shambhala Publications, 2009), 49.

5. Dalai Lama, "10 Questions for the Dalai Lama," *Time*, June 14, 2010, http://content.time.com/time/magazine/article/0,9171,1993865,00.html.

Chapter 14

1. Edwin A. M. Gale, "The Rise of Childhood Type 1 Diabetes in the 20th Century," *Diabetes* 51, no. 12 (December 2002): 3353–3361.

2. Dean Ornish et al., "Changes in Prostate Gene Expression in Men Undergoing an Intensive Nutrition and Lifestyle Intervention," *Proceedings of the National Academy of Sciences USA* 105, no. 24 (June 2008): 8369–8374.

Chapter 15

1. Johns Hopkins University Bloomberg School of Public Health, "US Autism Rate Unchanged in New CDC Report: Researchers Say It's Too Early to. Tell If Rate Has Stabilized," ScienceDaily, March 31, 2016, www.science-daily.com/releases/2016/03/160331154247.htm.

2. Ingmar Skoog et al., "Decreasing Prevalence of Dementia in 85-Year-Olds Examined 22 Years Apart: The Influence of Education and Stroke," *Scientific Reports* 7, no. 6136 (2017).

3. F. B. Hu et al., "Frequent Nut Consumption and Risk of Coronary Heart Disease in Women: Prospective Cohort Study," *BMJ* 317, no. 7169 (November 14, 1998): 1341–1345.

4. Jae Kwang Kim and Sang Un Park, "Current Potential Health Benefits of Sulforaphane," *EXCLI Journal* 15 (October 13, 2016): 571–577. DOI: 10.17179/excli2016-485.

5. Parris M. Kidd, Ph.D., "Glutathione: Systemic Protectant Against Oxidative and Free Radical Damage," *Alternative Medicine Review* 2, no. 3 (1997): 155–176.

6. Jeffrey D. Peterson et al., "Glutathione Levels in Antigen-Presenting Cells Modulate Th1 Versus Th2 Response Patterns," *Proceedings of the National Academy of Sciences USA* 95, no. 6 (March 17, 1998): 3071–3076.

7. Jess Gomez, "New Research Finds Routine Periodic Fasting Is Good for Your Health, and Your Heart," Intermountain Healthcare, April 3, 2011, http://intermountainhealthcare.org/about/careers/working/news/pages/home.aspx?NewsID=71.

Chapter 18

1. Mikhail V. Blagosklonny, "Why Human Lifespan Is Rapidly Increasing: Solving 'Longevity Riddle' with 'Revealed Slow Aging' Hypothesis," *Aging* (Albany NY) 2, no. 4 (April 2010): 177–182. DOI: 10.18632/aging.100139.

2. J. Gallinetti, E. Harputlugil, and J. R. Mitchell, "Amino Acid Sensing in Dietary-Restriction-Mediated Longevity: Roles of Signal-Transducing Kinases GCN2 and TOR," *Biochemical Journal* 449, no. 1 (January 1, 2013): 1–10. DOI: 10.1042/BJ20121098.

3. Bodo C. Melnik, "Leucine Signaling in the Pathogenesis of Type 2 Diabetes and Obesity," *World Journal of Diabetes* 3, no. 3 (March 15, 2012): 38–53. DOI: 10.4239/wjd.v3.i3.38.

4. Rainer J. Klement and Ulrike Kämmerer, "Is There a Role for Carbohydrate Restriction in the Treatment and Prevention of Cancer?," *Nutrition & Metabolism* 8 (2011): 75. DOI: 10.1186/1743-7075-8-75.

5. S. Yusuf et al., "Effect of Potentially Modifiable Risk Factors Associated with Myocardial Infarction in 52 Countries (the INTERHEART Study): Case-Control Study," *Lancet* 364, no. 9438 (September 11–17, 2004): 937–52.

6. The Nutrition Source, What Should I Eat? "Vegetables and Fruits," Harvard T.H. Chan School of Public Health, https://www.hsph.harvard.edu/nutritionsource/what-should-you-eat/vegetables-and-fruits.

7. P. Knekt et al., "Serum Vitamin D and the Risk of Parkinson Disease," *Archives of Neurology* 67, no. 7 (July 2010): 808–811. DOI: 10.1001/archneurol.2010.120.

8. M.C. Morris et al., "Consumption of Fish and N-3 Fatty Acids and Risk of Incident Alzheimer Disease," *Archives of Neurology* 60, no. 7 (July 2003): 940–946.

9. "Burning More Calories Associated with Greater Gray Matter Volume in Brain, Reduced Alzheimer's Risk," UPMC/University of Pittsburgh Schools of the Health Sciences, March 11, 2016, http://www.upmc.com/media/NewsReleases/2016/Pages/gray-matter.aspx.

10. Penny Baron, "The 10 Most Important Blood Tests," *Life Extension Magazine*, May 2006, http://www.lifeextension.com/magazine/2006/5/report_blood/Page-01.

Conclusion

1. Joseph Campbell, *The Hero with a Thousand Faces* (Novato, CA: New World Library, 2008), 205.

2. Swami Nikhilananda, trans., *The Bhagavad Gita* (New York: Ramakrishna-Vivekananda Center, 1944), 77–78.

3. Jean-Louis Santini, "Are Brains Shrinking to Make Us Smarter?," *Discovery News*, February 6, 2011, https://phys.org/news/2011-02-brains-smarter.html.

4. Campbell, *Hero with a Thousand Faces*, 142.

ACKNOWLEDGMENTS

I would like to thank David Perlmutter, M.D., for repairing my brain after I thought I had lost my mind. Mark Hyman, M.D., helped me to heal my body and discover an extraordinary level of health after Western medicine had given up on me. My shaman teachers in the high Andes healed my soul, showed me the journey beyond death, and revealed the ways to boundless health. These old medicine men and women taught me to taste Infinity.

Patricia Gift at Hay House has been the best ally and support an author could imagine, and my editors Sally Mason-Swaab and Nicolette Salamanca Young were godsends.

And above all, my deepest gratitude to my wife, Marcela Lobos, medicine woman extraordinaire, who healed my heart and patiently loved me while I completed this book.

ABOUT THE AUTHOR

Alberto Villoldo, Ph.D., has trained as a psychologist and medical anthropologist, and has studied the healing practices of the Amazon and the Andean shamans for more than 25 years. While an adjunct professor at San Francisco State University, he founded the Biological Self-Regulation Laboratory to study how the brain creates psychosomatic health and disease. Convinced that the mind could create health, he left his laboratory and traveled to the Amazon to work with the medicine men and women of the rain forest and learn their healing methods and mythology.

Dr. Villoldo directs The Four Winds Society, where he trains individuals in the U.S. and Europe in the practice of shamanic energy medicine. He is the founder of the Light Body School, which has campuses in New York, California, and Germany. He also directs the Center for Energy Medicine in Chile, where he investigates and practices the neuroscience of enlightenment. Dr. Villoldo has written numerous best-selling books, including *Shaman, Healer, Sage; The Four Insights; Courageous Dreaming; One Spirit Medicine;* and *Power Up Your Brain.*

Website: www.thefourwinds.com

Hay House Titles of Related Interest

YOU CAN HEAL YOUR LIFE, the movie,
starring Louise Hay & Friends
(available as an online streaming video)
www.hayhouse.com/louise-movie

THE SHIFT, the movie,
starring Dr. Wayne W. Dyer
(available as an online streaming video)
www.hayhouse.com/the-shift-movie

♦♦♦

ENERGY STRANDS: The Ultimate Guide to Clearing the Cords That Are Constricting Your Life, by Denise Linn

SACRED POWERS: The Five Secrets to Awakening Transformation, by davidji

SHAMANISM MADE EASY: Awaken and Develop the Shamanic Force Within, by Christa Mackinnon

UNCHARTED: The Journey through Uncertainty to Infinite Possibility, by Colette Baron-Reid

WINDS OF SPIRIT: Ancient Wisdom Tools for Navigating Relationships, Health, and the Divine, by Renee Baribeau

All of the above are available at your local bookstore,
or may be ordered by contacting Hay House (see next page).

We hope you enjoyed this Hay House book. If you'd like to receive our online catalog featuring additional information on Hay House books and products, or if you'd like to find out more about the Hay Foundation, please contact:

Hay House, Inc., P.O. Box 5100, Carlsbad, CA 92018-5100
(760) 431-7695 or (800) 654-5126
(760) 431-6948 (fax) or (800) 650-5115 (fax)
www.hayhouse.com® • www.hayfoundation.org

◆◆◆

Published in Australia by: Hay House Australia Pty. Ltd.,
18/36 Ralph St., Alexandria NSW 2015
Phone: 612-9669-4299 • *Fax:* 612-9669-4144
www.hayhouse.com.au

Published in the United Kingdom by: Hay House UK, Ltd.,
The Sixth Floor, Watson House, 54 Baker Street, London W1U 7BU
Phone: +44 (0)20 3927 7290 • *Fax:* +44 (0)20 3927 7291
www.hayhouse.co.uk

Published in India by: Hay House Publishers India,
Muskaan Complex, Plot No. 3, B-2, Vasant Kunj, New Delhi 110 070
Phone: 91-11-4176-1620 • *Fax:* 91-11-4176-1630
www.hayhouse.co.in

◆◆◆

Access New Knowledge.
Anytime. Anywhere.

Learn and evolve at your own pace
with the world's leading experts.

www.hayhouseU.com

MEDITATE.
VISUALIZE.
LEARN.

Get the **Empower You**
Unlimited Audio *Mobile App*

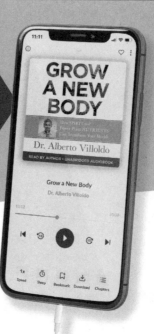

Get unlimited access to the entire Hay House audio library!

You'll get:

- 500+ inspiring and life-changing **audiobooks**

- 200+ ad-free **guided meditations** for sleep, healing, relaxation, spiritual connection, and more

- Hundreds of audios **under 20 minutes** to easily fit into your day

- **Exclusive content** *only* for subscribers

- **New audios** added every week

- No credits, **no limits**

Listen to the audio version of this book for FREE!

★★★★★ **I ADORE** this app.
I use it almost every day. Such a blessing. – Aya Lucy Rose

Scan me with your phone camera!

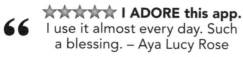

HAY HOUSE

TRY FOR FREE!
Go to: hayhouse.com/listen-free